The Essence of You

Your Guide to Gynecologic Health

Denise Howard, MD

Publisher Name: WAT-AGE Publishing
Legal Name: WAT-AGE Publishing LLC

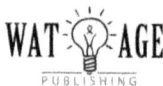

Softcover ISBN: 978-0-9906343-5-5
eBook ISBN: 978-0-9906343-6-2

Lulu Publishing Services rev. date: 07/27/2017

Table of Contents

Dedication

I'd like to express my gratitude to all the women I have cared for over the years: you have helped me be a better physician. This book is dedicated to you.

Introduction

When I was 12 years old, I discovered a blood stain in the lining of my panties. I was terrified. I grew up in a traditional working class southern family which meant that no one talked about private topics; as a result, I was quite the naïve adolescent. I wiped my vaginal area clean and prayed it would go away.

A short time later, when I went back to the bathroom to find that the bleeding had continued, I thought I was going to die of cancer. I worried about how I would tell my mother.

It took an hour to get up the nerve to speak to her. I remember she was deeply involved in her ironing and didn't immediately notice my tentative approach. I finally found the courage to speak, and I don't remember the words I used, but do remember stuttering because I was so scared. She didn't say anything, but instead turned and rummaged through a dresser drawer to retrieve a small booklet. She handed it to me and told me to read it. That was how I learned about the miracle of life. I was having my first period!

This experience wasn't the galvanizing event that made me decide to become a physician, but it did sensitize me to the importance of women and girls understanding their bodies. When I was a teenager I decided to become an obstetrician/gynecologist and never wavered from that decision. It was an appealing specialty for a variety of reasons; the main driver was the chance to be a primary health provider for women. Looking back, I am amazed that the decision I made based on reviewing various medical specialties in an encyclopedia are still valid after practicing for nearly 20 years.

The path to becoming a physician isn't an easy one, and this was especially true for me, an African American woman from a family with very limited resources. I worked hard and was fortunate to attend a state university. Later I was accepted into one of the top medical schools in the country, where I trained with some of the best physicians in America. Their influence, along with my humble upbringing, has helped me to be especially empathetic to the needs and perspective of my patients.

I have practiced medicine in the United States and internationally, and have taken care of women from a wide variety of economic, educational, ethnic, and religious backgrounds. Taking into consideration each woman's individual circumstance, I have consistently been struck by one thing: they all knew much less about their bodies and health than I would expect.

Limited understanding of health issues can significantly affect a woman's continued good health, as well as place her at the mercy of less-than-competent providers or an indifferent health care system. I continue to try to educate my patients about their health, bodies, and treatment options, but it is impossible to teach them everything they need to know in a short office visit. In addition, my influence has been limited to the women who visit me, and I want to reach so many more women and girls. That was my inspiration for writing this book, something that could be handed from one woman to another—and even from one generation to the next—that would educate women and girls about the health issues they may face over the course of their lives.

People who have a certain degree of health literacy make better health care decisions for themselves and their family. It is expected that physicians should play the role of educator as well as health care provider, but the reality is that, at present, comprehensive health education by physicians is an impossible expectation. Even physicians with the best intentions are trapped between trying to take care of as many patients as possible, generating enough revenue to cover their business expenses, and spending time with their families. Health care providers can't be solely responsible for their patients' health. Individuals must take responsibility for their own health and the health of their families. This process starts with health literacy.

Health literacy is defined as the degree to which an individual has the capacity to obtain, process, and understand basic health information to make appropriate health decisions. According to the National Assessment of Adult Literacy most people are at the basic or intermediate health literacy level. Only 12 percent of adults have proficient health literacy and 14 percent are below the basic level.[1] I certainly have witnessed this in the thousands and thousands of women I have cared for over the years.

Understanding health information gives people the skills to better navigate the health care system, helps them to take better care of themselves and their families, and aides them in making truly informed decisions when it comes to selecting treatment options. The objective of this book is to help improve every woman's health literacy by providing fundamental information that they can refer to over the years as health issues arise.

I have been blessed over my lifetime with so many opportunities to learn and grow. As a woman and a physician, the best way I can give back is to try to impart what I have learned to as many people as possible. I have designed this book to share my knowledge about routine gynecologic and women's health issues in a manner that is useful to women and girls. To make the book easier to navigate and understand, I decided to organize it by reproductive phase, with each section describing specific issues that may occur during this time. Each section is introduced with a personal story to emphasize the relevance of the condition under discussion. The names and stories do not refer to specific individuals but represent various interactions I have had with women over the years. A woman can read the sections that are relevant to her phase and/or condition, or the entire text as an overview. Use the book as a reference and share it with others.

Knowledge is indeed power, but when it comes to health, women have allowed others to be in control for far too long. In this current political climate, where restricting health access for women is acceptable in many circles, women need all the power they can get to take control of their health and that of their families. Women tend to make the health care decisions for their families. When women are better informed, their families are better off. This means that improving women's health is also in every man's best interest. This starts with increasing the health literacy for every woman, girl, and man. What you will read in *The Essence of You* is the first step to understanding your body and taking control of your health destiny.

Chapter 1

Uniquely You: Anatomy and Function

The human body truly is a masterpiece. The female form is phenomenal! Over the centuries, the female body has been exalted in art, music, and literature. From Indian nude bronzes of 2000 BC to the Aphrodite of fourth-century Greece, every culture has praised the female form. Even though the popular standards of beauty have changed over time, the celebration of the female body continues unabated.

The ability to conceive, bear, and nourish life distinguishes the female sex. To consider all the processes that must occur correctly to achieve this one goal is quite mind-boggling. Many of us take it for granted and do not give the proper respect to the complex, fragile gift that we have been given: LIFE! And even though some women choose not to reproduce, it is this potential that makes woman unique. To truly understand the gynecologic issues most women will face, we must start from this perspective; we must understand the reproductive process.

The first step to understanding gynecologic and other health problems is learning the names and the function of the female anatomy. Hopefully, with this knowledge, you will develop an appreciation and reverence for what is truly the essence of you. The ovaries, uterus, breast, vagina, fallopian tubes, and vulva are all the parts that make us different from men. Each serves a function and plays a role in the reproductive process. Each is susceptible to malfunction, malformation, dysfunction, and disease.

Every woman's body is beautiful and distinctive. Her breasts may be small or large, her hips narrow or wide, her waist slender or full. No matter what, you should celebrate your gift and never be ashamed. Take a mirror and examine every part of you, including your genital area. Never let anyone make you think it is ugly or unattractive. Get to know your body just as you know yourself. Treat it like the temple that it is. Most importantly, if you know yourself intimately you will be able to detect the early indications that something isn't right.

This chapter may be technically challenging to get through in one read, but the intent is for you to refer to it time and time again as you read through the whole book. I will also use medically correct terms to ensure a common language in discussing gynecologic health. This information is foundational and necessary to understanding the many health issues we will discuss in upcoming chapters. In addition, being able to use the correct terminology is important when communicating with your healthcare provider. I suggest that you review this chapter initially and then come back to it again if you read something in another chapter that is unclear.

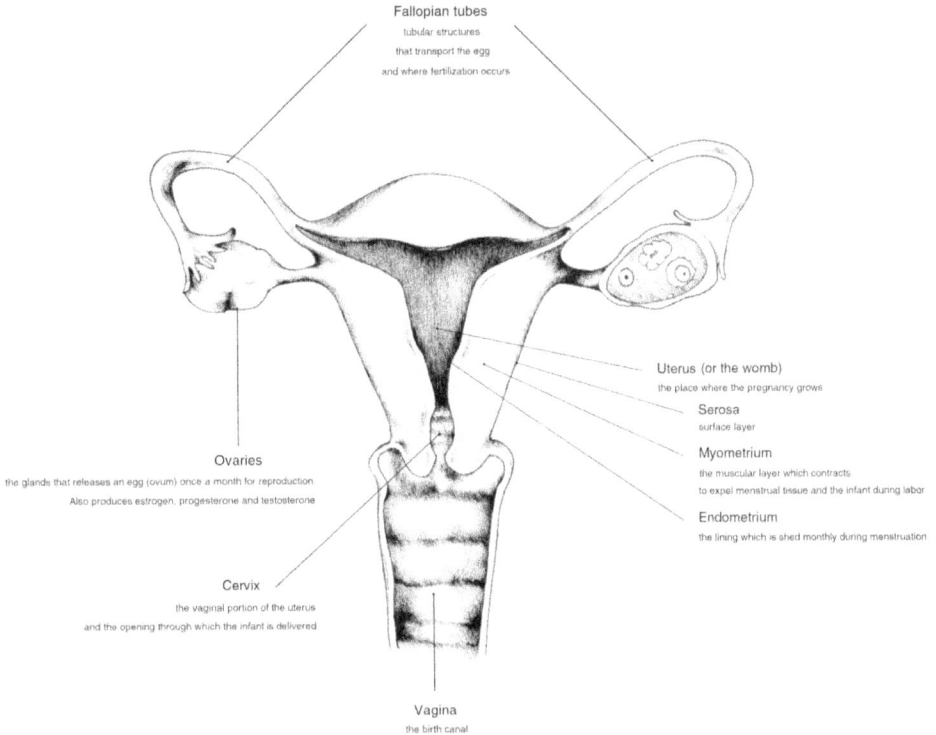

Fallopian tubes
tubular structures
that transport the egg
and where fertilization occurs

Uterus (or the womb)
the place where the pregnancy grows

Serosa
surface layer

Myometrium
the muscular layer which contracts
to expel menstrual tissue and the infant during labor

Endometrium
the lining which is shed monthly during menstruation

Ovaries
the glands that releases an egg (ovum) once a month for reproduction
Also produces estrogen, progesterone and testosterone

Cervix
the vaginal portion of the uterus
and the opening through which the infant is delivered

Vagina
the birth canal

The Organs

The **ovaries** are often the least discussed reproductive organs. They are, however, responsible for the most vital function that makes us distinctly woman. We give them little thought and don't appreciate their value until they are not functioning properly.

These twin organs are located in the pelvis, attached to the pelvic sidewall and uterus via structures called ligaments. Ovaries tend to be approximately 3 to 5 cm in diameter. They produce an egg once a month, typically taking turns making a single egg. It is unusual for both to release an egg in the same month, but if they do and the eggs are fertilized, the result is a set of fraternal twins.

In addition to producing eggs capable of being fertilized, the ovaries also produce hormones. These hormones are responsible for ovulation and sustaining an early pregnancy if conception occurs. The hormones produced include estrogen, progesterone, and testosterone. These hormones also contribute to emotional balance, daily energy, sexual desire, a regular sleep cycle, and probably many more functions that make us feel healthy and normal.

The **uterus,** or womb, is the organ where a fetus grows during pregnancy. The term "womb" is often used to invoke feelings of warmth and safety because this is how we imagine the fetus feels for the nine months it spends in the uterus developing. Of all the female organs, it is the one that has always been recognized as the site where the miracle of life occurs. This simple organ is emblematic of total security, complete acceptance, and unconditional love. It is no wonder it is the most hallowed of all our female organs.

The uterus is a muscular organ comprised of two parts: the main body—called the "corpus"—and the cervix. The cervix is the vaginal portion of the uterus and is the gateway to the womb. It's the part that stays closed to retain a growing pregnancy and, at the time of labor, gradually dilates to allow delivery of the fetus through the vagina.

The 6- to 8-centimeter-long corpus is made up predominantly of smooth muscle, but its cavity is lined with endometrial tissue that proliferates during the cycle and sheds at the time of menstruation. This lining, called the endometrium, has two layers: the functional layer that grows or proliferates to prepare for implantation of the fertilized egg (this is the layer that sheds if pregnancy does not occur) and the basal layer, which provides the base for regeneration of the functional layer when the cycle repeats itself in the absence of pregnancy. That is, it's the part that grows the blood-laden tissue that will shed off during menstruation. The outer portion of the uterus is covered with a membrane called the peritoneum and is called the serosal layer. Imagine an avocado sliced in half. The inner portion where the seed sits is the endometrium, the fleshy part that we eat is the myometrium, and the skin is the serosal layer.

The uterus sits between the bladder, located anteriorly (toward the front of the body), and the rectum (bowel), located posteriorly (toward the back of the body). The exact position varies from person to person. For some women, the uterus sits anteriorly and flexes toward the anterior abdomen; this is known as anteverted or anteflexed. In others, it sits more posteriorly and can literally lie on the rectum. This is called retroverted or retroflexed. In some women, it sits midway between the bladder and the rectum. Where and how it sits is irrelevant, just like the shape and tilt of the nose, though sometimes it can create a challenge for a gynecologist when trying to visualize the cervix during a pelvic examination. (Many times, I have had to get on my knees for a better view or ask my patient to grab her knees and pull them to her chest to move the cervix into view.) You shouldn't worry about this as it typically has no impact on your health.

The **fallopian tubes** are tubular structures that branch off the uterus at its dome and end in approximation to each ovary. The term "adnexae" refers to both the tube and ovary. They are approximately seven to 12 centimeters in length and have three portions: the isthmus, the ampulla, and the fimbria. The function of the tubes is to pick up the egg released by the ovary, provide a site for fertilization, and then nourish the fertilized egg and transport it to the uterus.

The **vagina** is a word many people are reluctant to utter. It is even a term that leads to blockage of certain internet sites when typed into a search engine. Rather than using the correct anatomical term, women prefer to give it intimate nicknames like 'kitty', 'vajayjay', 'pupusa', 'vaginald', 'pumpum' and many others. Vagina is the proper anatomical name for this part of the female body and you should not be embarrassed to use this term. No matter how you chose to refer to it, please appreciate it as one element that makes you uniquely woman.

The vaginal orifice is the opening to the **vagina**, the site of copulation. The vagina, also known as the birth canal, is a fibromuscular tube that attaches to the pelvic sidewall. It receives lubrication from fluid secreted from the cervix and Bartholin's gland. The epithelium is colonized with a mixture of bacteria that maintains a neutral pH balance. Vaginas accommodate the penis during intercourse and hold the semen, providing time for the sperm to travel through the cervix. It is the passage through which the fetus travels during delivery, once the cervix is completely dilated.

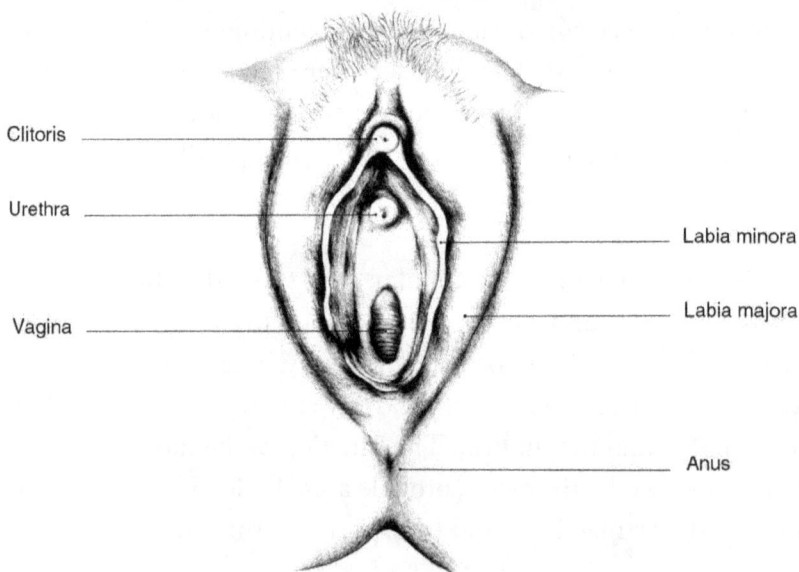

The **vulva**—from the Latin, meaning wrapper or covering—consists of the mons pubis, labia majora, labia minora, clitoris, and the vaginal and urethral orifices. The mons pubis is the hair-bearing region over the pubic bone. The labia majora is the hair-covered skin fold on either side of the labia minora. It is like the leaves of a flower, while the labia minora, a thinner fold of hairless tissue that lies between the labia majora and the vaginal opening, is akin to its petals. These structures are sometimes described as the outer and inner vaginal "lips."

The **clitoris** is the female equivalent of the penis in that it is a highly sensitive, nerve-filled erectile structure. This is the center of orgasmic activity for most women. It is also one of the lesser understood organs of the female anatomy, though an important one for a variety of reasons, both physical and psychological.

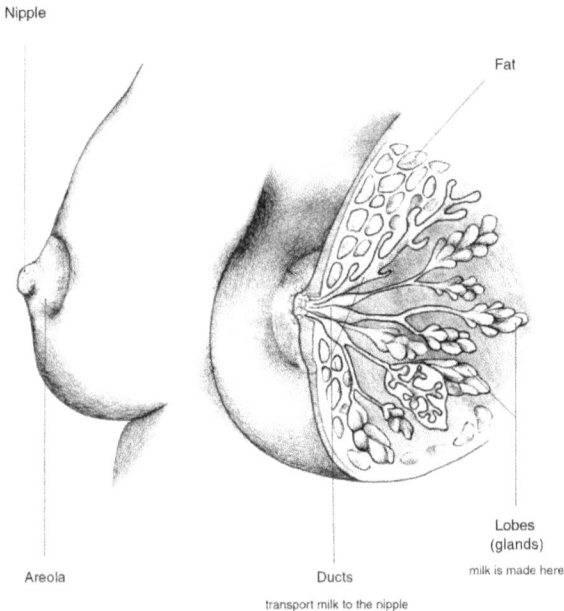

Nipple

Fat

Lobes
(glands)
milk is made here

Areola

Ducts

transport milk to the nipple

Breasts

Mammary organs that are designed to produce milk and transport it to the suckling infant

The breasts are the female organs that distinctly identify woman. They tend to be the focus of much attention and some women invest great effort in ensuring their attributes are perfectly emphasized. And like the vagina, they are also treated familiarly, given nicknames like 'boobs', 'the girls', 'tits', 'puppies', 'my friends', 'knockers' and many more. They are probably the most celebrated organs of the female body but no matter the shape or size, the function is the same.

Breasts are paired mammary organs that function to produce milk and transport it to a suckling infant. They are composed of fibrous and fat tissue that surrounds 15 to 20 lobes of glands. The lobes form a circle around the nipple and communicate with the nipple via ducts that allow the passage of milk. The areola is the darker, thicker, more wrinkled skin that extends 1 to 2 centimeters out from the nipples onto the skin of the breast. The areolar and nipples are designed to fit into the mouth of a suckling infant, facilitating milk let-down.

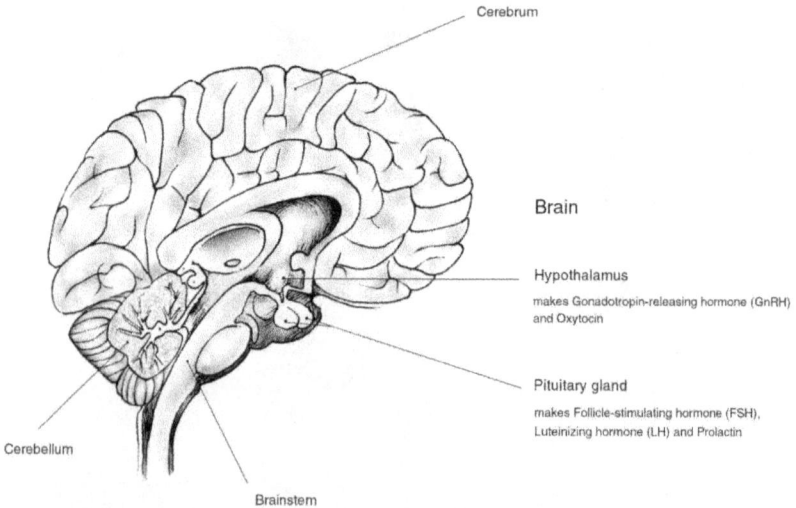

Cerebrum

Brain

Hypothalamus
makes Gonadotropin-releasing hormone (GnRH) and Oxytocin

Pituitary gland
makes Follicle-stimulating hormone (FSH), Luteinizing hormone (LH) and Prolactin

Cerebellum

Brainstem

Communicating Chemicals: The Hormones

Hormones are substances that are secreted by one organ that travels in the blood stream to another organ, telling that particular organ to perform a specific action. Hormones and other substances called neurotransmitters are a mechanism for communication. There are certain hormones that play a specific role in reproductive processes.

The expression, raging hormones isn't a joke. This describes exactly how some women feel a week or two before menstruation or during the transition to menopause. Fluctuating hormone levels contribute to the runner's high and the postpartum lows. Our mood and mental outlook can be seriously affected by hormone levels, which can cause mood swings, depression, low energy, and even angry outbursts. Not every woman is affected in the same manner and many don't notice the changes in the hormonal levels during the ovulatory cycle but for those seriously impacted, help is available. But what are they exactly?

Estrogens are hormones that are produced by the ovary. They are also produced in other tissue. There are three major types: estrone, estradiol, and estriol. Estradiol is the major product of ovarian production. All three are produced at even higher rates during pregnancy.

Estrogen stimulates the uterine lining to grow or proliferate in preparation for implantation of a fertilized egg. The site on the ovary where the egg is released is called the corpus luteum. It continues to produce estrogen in greater amounts after ovulation.

Progesterone is produced by the corpus luteum as well. The amount produced is less than 1 milligram per day prior to ovulation but after ovulation it increases ten-fold. Continued secretion sustains the endometrium, thereby supporting continued development of a pregnancy. It is produced in even higher doses by the placenta which takes over complete production of progesterone by 10 weeks of pregnancy.

Follicle-stimulating hormone (FSH) is secreted in the region of the brain called the pituitary gland and travels to the ovary where it exerts its effects. It stimulates growth of the ovarian follicles. This occurs at the beginning of the menstrual cycle.

Luteinizing hormone (LH) is secreted in the region of the brain called the pituitary gland and travels to the ovary where it exerts its effects. Its sudden release causes the expulsion of an egg from the dominant follicle. This is called ovulation.

Gonadotropin-releasing hormone (GnRH) is released in the brain in a region called the hypothalamus. It controls release of the gonadotropins, FSH and LH. GnRH is secreted in a pulsatile fashion which in turn regulates the production and secretion of those gonadotropins.

Oxytocin is produced in the region of the brain called the hypothalamus. It causes contraction of the uterine muscles, which results in labor. It also leads to contraction of breast duct cells and subsequent milk let down. Its release is triggered by nipple stimulation which typically occurs with suckling.

Prolactin is formed in the region of the brain called the pituitary gland. It instructs the breast to make milk. Breast stimulation by the suckling infant leads to increased levels of prolactin, resulting in continued milk production by the breast.

Putting It All Together: What Makes a Woman a Woman

There are three reproductive related functions that are unique to the female: **menstruation, gestation and lactation.** In addition, there is a reproductive-related event that has a dramatic effect on the longevity and quality of a woman's life: **menopause**. Understanding these normal events is the key to understanding the problems that can arise during different stages of a woman's life.

Menstruation: Is it a blessing or a curse? For many women, the monthly appearance of this "crimson wave" is reassurance that they are not pregnant. For others, it is reassurance that they are still able to get pregnant. Some women see it as a monthly nuisance and others view it as a disrupting, painful, unwelcome event. In this day and age, it doesn't have to be either. Medical advances have made it possible to avoid the physical and emotional distress that it brings until pregnancy is desired. But before you manipulate it, you should understand it.

What causes the monthly menstruation?

Menstruation is the monthly shedding of the endometrium when pregnancy does not occur. The first day of bleeding represents Day 1 of the cycle. There are two phases of the endometrial cycle: proliferative and secretory.

The proliferative phase is associated with ovarian follicle growth and the increased secretion of estrogen. Estrogen causes the functional layer of the endometrium to regrow.

The secretory phase starts after ovulation has occurred. Estrogen and progesterone act on the endometrium to stabilize it in preparation for implantation if fertilization occurs. This happens around 7 days post ovulation.

If implantation does not occur, the corpus luteum (cystic structure on ovary that appears at the site of ovulation) will involute leading to a drop in the production of estrogen and progesterone. The endometrium starts to shed resulting in menstruation. This typically occurs around day 28. The cessation of menses is a complex process. The return of estrogen production by the new developing follicles in the ovary is a major factor.

How does pregnancy occur?

Follicle stimulating hormone (FSH) tells the ovaries to begin follicle development. Many follicles compete to be "the one". Estrogen levels increase. A sudden increase in luteinizing hormone leads to the release of one egg (and sometimes two). This is called ovulation. The site of the released egg becomes the corpus luteum. The corpus luteum secretes estrogen and progesterone.

Imagine that each month, out of the hundreds of thousands of dormant eggs in the ovary, only one is released, that one has a low probability of being fertilized, and that fertilized egg has a low chance of developing into a normal pregnancy. This complex process results in a truly unique and highly resilient infant.

Sperm contained within the ejaculate of the male travel rapidly through the cervix. The transportation occurs via a combination of the swimming action of the sperm and uterine contractions. In general, 200 to 300 million sperm are contained in the semen but only 200 actually make it to the fallopian tube. This can happen as early as 80 hours after ejaculation. Of this 200, only one is strong enough, fast enough, and healthy enough to fertilize the egg. Just think about it: The Olympiad-level eggs and sperms compete to be allowed the privilege of conception. Your child is the product of the best of the best. The gold-medal egg and gold-medal sperm join forces to give you an off spring. What an award!

The egg reaches the fallopian tube two to three minutes after ovulation. It is grasped by the tubal fimbria and moved through the tube by tubal contraction. Fertilization occurs within 12 to 24 hours of ovulation. If two eggs are fertilized, then fraternal twins result. Once a sperm penetrates the egg, the now-fertilized egg can now start to duplicate, developing into a mass of cells that will eventually develop into the embryo. If for some reason this mass of cells separates into two distinct bunches, identical twins will develop. The fertilized embryo will travel another two to three days within the fallopian tube until it reaches the endometrium.

The embryo enters the uterus on day 18 or 19 of the cycle. Implantation occurs on day 21 or 22 of the cycle, which is 5 to 7 days after fertilization. The embryo adheres to the wall of the endometrium and burrows in.

How is milk produced?

An increased estrogen level causes an increased production of prolactin in the maternal pituitary gland. Prolactin is the hormone that stimulates the growth of breast tissue, but only colostrum is produced during pregnancy. Progesterone inhibits further milk production.

An abrupt decrease in estrogen and progesterone after delivery of the fetus leads to milk production in the breast. Secretion into the breast gland ducts occur three to four days post-delivery. Suckling causes an even greater increase in prolactin production, which is required to initiate and continue milk production. This suckling also causes secretion of oxytocin, a hormone that is known for producing feelings of love and attachment, which also leads to contraction of the breast cells and emptying of the ducts. A breast can store milk for 48 hours before production decreases in the absence of suckling. Discontinuation of suckling is all that is required to stop lactation.

What happens that leads to menopause?

Menopause is the result of ovarian failure defined as that point in time when permanent cessation of menstruation occurs. The average age of menopause is 51.3 years, but can range from 45 to 55 years of age. In the past, this change was viewed as a death knell, but of course this was perspective of a society that said a woman's only value was in her ability to reproduce. Thankfully, times have changed. With a life expectancy of almost 80 years, many women view this transition as liberating. Suddenly they are free of all the restraints monthly menstruation brings.

Perimenopause is the period surrounding menopause where ovarian function is slowing and ovulation is less frequent. The menstrual cycle length increases. This tends to occur after age 40 and can continue for two to eight years before the actual menopause.

Hormone levels reflect these changes. FSH levels tend to be increased. This hormone is working harder and harder to get the ovary to make follicles. The remaining follicles tend to be less responsive so higher levels of FSH are required to stimulate them. This explains the decreased fertility in this age group. The estrogen levels tend to remain the same during this period. At the point that there are no follicles left to respond, menstruation ceases.

After menopause, there is a significant increase in follicle stimulating and luteinizing hormones. Estrogen and testosterone levels are also much less but production in other sites occur. It is the low estrogen levels that cause many of the bothersome symptoms of menopause.

THE BOTTOM LINE

- The ovaries produce estrogens. Ovarian failure or removal of the ovaries result in menopause.
- The purpose of the uterus is to provide an environment for the growth and nourishment of the fetus. It is a vehicle of reproduction and has no known purpose once this mission is complete.
- The monthly period is the shedding endometrium. Its purpose is to provide a nesting site in which the fertilized egg can implant and grow.

- Chemicals from the brain tell the ovaries to produce an egg each month and to make hormones. The hormones from the ovaries communicate with the endometrium, directing it to shed or to maintain its lining in the presence of a pregnancy.

Chapter 2

The Adolescent Years: The Awakening

Parents take pride in watching their child develop and each stage introduces a different set of concerns. This is especially true when signs of sexual development occur. This marks the realization that their princess is no longer a baby and presents a whole host of new worries. A child goes through so many changes during this life phase and understanding the process is the best weapon to help parents and girls navigate this wondrous, yet potentially frightening period.

Adolescence is the developmental stage when a girl starts to develop sexual characteristics. At this point hormonal changes are occurring that lead to breast development and that reflect the awakening of the previously quiescent ovaries.

Gynecologic issues that arise during this time typically are related to the menstrual cycle. Most adolescents are not sexually active yet, so issues related to this will be addressed in the next chapter, on young adulthood. One of the greatest health risks to adolescents, however, relates to sexual abuse, and we will address that subject in this chapter.

It is extremely important to remember that, despite the development of secondary sexual characteristics that are the preamble to adulthood, adolescents are still children, and it is the duty of the parent or other custodian to protect and guide them through this exciting and potentially challenging time.

Adults are responsible for making health decisions for their children. Part of this is preventive health care, which includes routine childhood vaccinations. Recent discussions of the pros and cons of regular vaccinations have highlighted concerns parents have about the long-term effect of this intervention, but one thing is certain: Vaccinations have been proven to be effective in preventing previously life-threatening infectious illnesses. There isn't any scientific evidence to support the notion that vaccines cause autism or contribute to any other developmental problems. Vaccines save lives and are undeniably the greatest medical breakthrough of all time. Now there is even one that is effective against a virus known to cause cervical cancer.

This chapter will discuss sexual development, menstrual related problems, sexual abuse, and human papilloma virus prevention.

Sexual Development

Anna comes to see me every year for her routine gynecologic exam. When I see her, I can't believe a whole year has passed. While reviewing her medical file, and getting an update on other health-related issues, I ask about her kids. It is always heartwarming to hear about the antics of her young children, especially because I delivered them. She usually has some funny stories to tell, but this time she pauses and says, "Doctor, my little girl isn't so little anymore." I pause what I am doing and ask her to explain. She has noticed that her 9-year-old daughter has started to develop hair in her arm pits. She knows that this is a sign of sexual development but is unsure of the sequence of events and therefore can't tell her daughter what to expect next. After finishing her examination and making sure she has everything she needs, I take a few minutes to explain puberty and make some suggestions to help her and her daughter become comfortable with this transition.

Puberty is that period when a person first becomes capable of reproduction, usually occurring between the ages of 10 and 16 years. These changes generally take, on average, four and a half years from beginning to completion. Factors that play a role in the timing of sexual development include genetics, nutrition, health, geographic location, and exposure to light.

Puberty is triggered by the increase in female hormones, which drive the development of "secondary sexual characteristics," such as hair growth in the arm pits or pelvic area. The sequence of events typically starts when the body resumes production of GnRH (Gonadotropin-releasing hormone), which has been suppressed since birth. This leads to an increase in the production of luteinizing hormone (LH) and follicle stimulating hormone (FSH), and a subsequent increase in an estrogen called estradiol.

Estradiol is responsible for breast development, fat distribution, and growth of the vagina and uterus. Skeletal growth also occurs during this time. There is an increase in androgen production by the adrenal gland, which causes the hair growth in the pubic region and under the arms. At some point, there is enough estrogen production to stimulate and grow the endometrium (lining of the uterus), at which point the first menses or period occurs.

Pubic and axillary (arm pit) hair typically starts to grow between the ages of 8 and 10. This results from increased production of androgens (usually described as male hormones) by the adrenal gland. This typically occurs two years before the onset of menstruation.

Breast development starts right after the pubertal growth spurt, typically around 10 years of age. After breast development, but just before the onset of menses, there is a period of accelerated growth, usually doubling in 1 year. The onset of menstruation is the last event of pubertal development and occurs in most girls at 12.8 years with a range of 9 to 18 years of age.

Ovulation (release of an egg) typically does not occur right away, and can often take up to 12 or 18 months after the first menses. Thus, girls can experience irregular or heavy bleeding during menstruation. Between 25 and 50 percent of adolescents experience up to four years of this irregular bleeding after the first period but before ovulation occurs. [1]

During this adolescent period, there is a rapid increase in bone density that also occurs. For some reason the increase in bone density is greater in some groups compared to others. In either case this increase in skeletal mass can be aided by calcium intake. This provides a window of opportunity to facilitate skeletal health and hopefully minimize the risk of Osteoporosis. This explains the rationale behind the traditional emphasis on drinking your milk. It is important to include an adequate amount of calcium in the diet of developing girls to maximize their bone development.

THE BOTTOM LINE

- Sexual development takes place over several years.
- This is a crucial time for bone development. Calcium consumption is important to maximize bone density and to prevent Osteoporosis later in life.
- Awareness of sexuality is occurring. This is the time to discuss the body changes and explain menstruation.
- Girls can get pregnant at this point if sexual exposure occurs.

Menstrual Related Problems

The most common gynecologic problems young girls experience is usually related to menstruation. Typical complaints relate to irregular, frequent, or heavy bleeding. Problems related to the onset of the period are described below. This can be a stressful time for both the parent and the child but also exciting as the girl embarks on the journey to womanhood.

Early Onset of Menses or "Precocious Puberty"

I rush into my office for a consult visit with a new patient. She is the first patient of the day and I am running late after taking longer than expected to see my post-surgical patient who is still in the hospital. I open my mouth to apologize and am taken aback when I see Rita, an established patient of mine that I had just seen the previous week. She rises when I come in, "Hi Dr. Howard, I know you are surprised to see me but I need your advice." Sitting next to her is a young girl I haven't seen before. I smile immediately and take a seat. Rita introduces me to her 8-year-old daughter, Nina, and explains that she started her period last week. It terrified Nina and was the last thing Rita expected. Rita is concerned that this is much too early and is worried that there must be something medically wrong.

The early onset of menses is called "precocious puberty." Puberty is described as premature if there is the appearance of sexual characteristics before the age of 8. Sexual characteristics include the onset of menses, the appearance of pubic or axillary hair or breast development. These characteristics can appear alone or in the usual expected series as explained earlier.

There are many potential causes for precocious puberty. Most of the time a cause can't be identified and the girl can expect to have a normal reproductive life. However, it's important to see a doctor because other potential causes could include an ovarian tumor, a brain tumor, abnormal production of specific hormones, and problems of the thyroid or adrenal glands.

The most important step in determining the cause—or lack of cause—is to see a health care provider. Sometimes a referral to a specialist such as an endocrinologist or a reproductive endocrinologist may be necessary. Though cases like those are rare, it is crucial to rule out any possible life-threatening cause.

If there isn't an underlying medical problem, then the final consideration becomes the consequence of early puberty. The major potential consequence is stunted growth.

Approximately 50 percent of girls with precocious puberty will attain an adult height of less than 5 feet.[2] The presence of estrogen results in early closure of the boney growth plates. Other concerns relate to the appearance of sexual maturity in an individual who is still emotionally and intellectually a child, as well as the risk of pregnancy in the case of sexual exposure.

There is a way to stop this early development. Medications described as GnRH agonists can stop the sexual maturation process, and even reverse some of the signs of puberty. It is like the GnRH hormone produced in the hypothalamus gland, which is normally delivered at regular intervals to stimulate the production of the pituitary hormones (LH and FSH). When given as a treatment, the body sees a constant dose and this blocks the production of LH and FSH. It is administered as a monthly or quarterly injection that suppresses the hormones involved in sexual development. The treatment can be stopped at an appropriate time, allowing for continuation of development. This has the advantage of allowing the continuation of normal bone development and the final attainment of the intended adult height.

I referred Rita and Nina to a reproductive endocrinologist for a consultation. This subspecialist manages issues related to female reproduction and development and should be able to do a comprehensive evaluation, explain management options, and provide the most current treatments, if needed. I try to stay current on most gynecologic treatments but recognize that it is impossible to know everything. The hallmark of a good doctor is one who knows when to ask for help and who makes decisions that are in the best interest of their patients—even when it means turning over that care to someone with more expertise.

Late Onset of Menses, or "Delayed Puberty"

A few days later I saw a girl whose problem was the exact opposite of Nina's. Jessie was sitting in my office when I entered for the last visit of a busy day. I introduced myself and shook her hand. She explained that her dad was in the waiting room because she preferred to see me alone but said I should explain everything to him when the visit was over. (This mature kid immediately made me feel comfortable. It's supposed to be the other way around!) She quickly explained the reason for her visit: She had been stuffing tissue in her bra to give the appearance of having breasts and pretending to her friends that she had a monthly menstruation. She was too embarrassed to admit that she had not started her period, but now that she had turned 16 she was worried that something was wrong.

I told Jessie I was certain that she was normal and that a small percentage of girls develop at a later age. To reassure her, I ordered some simple blood tests and a pelvic ultrasound and pointed out her uterus and ovaries on the ultrasound images. I then explained the blood test results, which showed that her hormone levels were in the range of someone who had not yet gone through puberty. I advised her to come back to see me in a year.

One is considered to have delayed puberty if there are no signs of sexual characteristics by age 17. This is a rare occurrence, and the causes can be varied. A thorough evaluation by a specialist is recommended to identify the cause and to provide needed medical intervention in some cases.

Ovarian failure is the cause 43 percent of the time; 26 percent of the time the cause is an abnormality in the development of the reproductive tract. In 13 percent of cases a defect in hormone production in the pituitary or hypothalamus gland is responsible, or a tumor in the brain is identified. The reason for delayed puberty can be treatable in 18 percent of cases. Normal physiologic delay, extreme weight loss, thyroid disorder, benign tumors of the pituitary gland, and other endocrine disorders can lead to delayed puberty.[2]

<u>Irregular and Heavy Menstrual Bleeding</u>

One aspect of my practice is taking call. This means being available for 24 hours or more to take care of emergencies. I was asked by the in-house doctor to come see a patient named Brandy who had been admitted for severe anemia. I arrived on the unit and logged in to the electronic system to review the health record. I noted the patient was 14 years old. I found a pale girl with wide brown eyes staring at me as I walked through the door. I gave her a big smile and introduced myself as Dr. Denise. Wanting to make her comfortable I attempted to interject some humor by asking her, "What's a lovely girl such as yourself doing in a place like this?" I rolled my eyes and glanced around the room trying to be as dramatic as possible. She giggled and explained. It seemed she has had irregular periods since starting them at age 12. She recently skipped four months (more than usual) and now has been bleeding for three weeks straight. She had fainted so her mom brought her straight to the emergency department. She was admitted and given a blood transfusion. Now she was feeling better but was worried that this might occur again.

As mentioned in the section on sexual development, close to half of adolescents can take up to four years to ovulate consistently. The potential consequence of not ovulating is heavy and irregular bleeding.

If an egg is not released, progesterone—a hormone that counteracts the effect of estrogen on the endometrium (the lining of the uterus that is shed monthly)—is not produced. Lack of progesterone results in continued growth of the endometrium. At some point, it starts to break down spontaneously. This occurs in isolated areas and is not simultaneous or synchronous. Once one area stops bleeding another area may start. This bleeding can go on for days or even weeks.

Not only is this annoying and disruptive, it can also be life-threatening. Severe anemia can result in dizziness, weakness, fainting, shortness of breath, and fatigue. Heart attack and stroke can even occur in rare extreme cases.

Thankfully, hormonal therapy is readily available and effective. A combination of estrogen and progestin therapy, a formulation typically found in birth control pills, can stop acute bleeding. When given daily it can regulate the menstrual cycle to prevent recurrent and excessive bleeding. Therapies using progestin, the synthetic version of a woman's own progesterone, can also be given alone, either daily or 10-12 days each month. It counteracts the effect of estrogen and allows for a controlled endometrial shedding. GnRH agonist therapy is also available in cases where the patient does not respond to the oral hormone therapy.

<u>Painful Periods or Dysmenorrhea</u>

I had a non-stop morning of patients and my afternoon schedule was equally full. I was almost done eating a desperately needed sandwich when my front office manager came into the break room and thrust the phone at me, "Would you please talk to this woman named Cindi?" I had worked with my staff long enough to know when I needed to just follow orders, so I took the phone and introduced myself. "Thank God! You are there!" The anxious voice on the other end shouted. I reassured her that I was and asked how I could help. She explained that she had just picked her daughter up from school because the daughter was experiencing the worst period of her life, mainly due to pain. She needed some advice and apologized for calling but they had not received their insurance cards yet and she really wanted to avoid an unnecessary emergency visit if at all possible.

Her daughter had missed school in the past because of the pain but this seemed worse than usual.

The pain that occurs with menstruation is described as a cramping sensation in the lower abdomen, pelvis, and back. The notorious "cramps" can be experienced by 60-72% of adolescents and young women. A substance called prostaglandin is released by the endometrium. This substance causes the muscles of the uterus to squeeze or contract. This is perceived as the painful cramps of menstruation. Other annoying symptoms include nausea, vomiting, headaches, and diarrhea, the consequences being missed school and work and the inability to participate in other planned activities.

Use of nonsteroidal anti-inflammatory drugs (NSAIDs) such as ibuprofen and naproxen are effective in decreasing the sensation of pain in most cases, and there are many other drugs in this category that are equally effective. If these methods do not help, then the other treatment option is a combined estrogen and progestin medication that comes in the form of a birth control pill. This method is extremely effective and makes a great difference in the quality of life during the time of the period. There is no need for a girl or women to suffer needlessly.

THE BOTTOM LINE

- Precocious puberty typically has no long-term health consequences.
- Delayed puberty is a rare occurrence.
- Heavy irregular bleeding may continue to be a problem for up to four years after the onset of menses.
- Nonsteroidal anti-inflammatory drugs work for menstrual cramps.

Sexual Abuse

I was just about to exit the auditorium doors after giving a health talk to a group of middle school girls when I noticed a shy girl hovering near the exit. "Hi," I said stopping to give her a chance to talk. She told me her name was Danielle and she wanted to talk to a doctor about her friend, Eva. Apparently, Eva was very uncomfortable around her mother's new boyfriend but didn't know how to tell her mom. It seemed that the boyfriend had become too friendly and was even touching her in inappropriate places. Eva was afraid to be alone with him but didn't know what to do. Situations like this are quite difficult but must be addressed. I advised her to urge her friend Eva to talk to her mom or any other adult she felt comfortable with. I also made sure Danielle had my contact information and that of other support services so she would have some resource in the event of an emergency.

Unfortunately, this is a seldom discussed but very common problem. Approximately 44% percent of women report that they have been the victim of some type of sexual violence during their lifetime. Forty percent of women have been sexually assaulted before the age of 18. Eight percent of girls experience a rape or attempted rape and more than 90% of these victims know the perpetrator.[3,4] These are disturbing statistics!

Violent crime and aggression toward women is strikingly underreported, for many reasons. Embarrassment, fear of retribution, and disbelief that the perpetrator will be punished are the most common ones. The reporting of crimes against children is dependent on the guardians' knowledge and concern.

There are both immediate and long-term health threats after sexual assault. Death, mutilation, and physical injury are the more extreme examples, as are exposure to sexually transmitted infections and risk of pregnancy.

The long-term consequences are typically emotional, psychological, and behavioral. Children who have been sexually abused are statistically more likely to run away from home, become involved in prostitution and substance abuse, and participate in other criminal activity. Many will suffer from low self-esteem, leading to multiple sexual partners or becoming involved in abusive relationships. They are at a higher risk of depression, suicide, chronic pain syndromes, and sexual dysfunction.

This represents a crisis. We should be doing a better job of protecting our children, our future.

I followed up with Danielle a few days later and learned that Eva didn't exist. She was referring to herself. Danielle had taken my advice and gotten up the courage to talk to her mother. Her mom was horrified to hear Danielle's experience with her new boyfriend and immediately broke off the relationship. She made Danielle promise to always come to her with any problems and made a point of saying that Danielle was the most important person in her life.

Not all victims of sexual abuse are as fortunate as Danielle to have such a supportive relationship. For those who are at risk or have suffered from sexual assault, there are many other ways to protect girls from abuse. Physicians, teachers, religious leaders and other family members are potential sources of support if a child feels comfortable reaching out to these individuals. Health care providers in the United States are legally obligated to report suspected cases of abuse to the authorities. Resources are available to assist children at risk, and local hospitals that provide emergency services to women and children will know how to get in touch with support services in their area.

THE BOTTOM LINE

- It is the parent's or custodian's responsibility to be a better protector of their children:
- Be more vigilant in monitoring what they do and who they are with.
- Be cautious in choosing adults to supervise your children.
- Don't place your child in vulnerable situations.
- Talk to your child about the fact that bad things can happen, about not being overly trusting of adults, and about stranger avoidance.
- Make sure your child is comfortable speaking to you about any concern.
- Situations to approach with caution:

1. Spending the night at others' homes.
2. Large events or places where the child might be unsupervised, such as parties, the mall, sporting events, and airport.
3. School events that are chaperoned by teachers and coaches.
4. Scheduled extracurricular activities, such as private music lessons or practices.
5. Boyfriends (of the mother) or relatives who seek out opportunities to be alone with your child.
6. Overeager or overzealous individuals who want to help because they just love kids so much.

Human Papilloma Virus (HPV) Prevention

Karen, one of my nurse colleagues, stopped me during rounds one morning to ask my opinion of the HPV vaccine. Her pediatrician advised her to give her teenage daughter the HPV vaccine but Karen has her doubts. She had heard that it could cause problems and many of her friends from the neighborhood and church think it's a bad idea. She wanted to do everything she could to protect her daughter and didn't know if giving her the vaccine was the right thing to do. We've worked together for years, so she trusted my opinion.

The adolescent period provides a unique opportunity to prevent one of the deadliest cancers, cervical cancer. Cervical cancer is a malignancy of the cervix which is known to result from sexual exposure to a virus called Human Papilloma Virus (HPV). Once the cells of the cervix are infected, it is possible for the body to fight the infection. However, in some cases the cervix may undergo precancerous changes and eventually develop cancer. This process can take 10 or more years. These viruses can also cause malignancies of the vulva, vagina, anus, and penis, as well as a condition called recurrent respiratory papillomatosis. **See Chapter 8 to learn more about cervical cancer prevention.**

Chapter 3

Young Adulthood: The Genesis

This is the period when a girl transitions to womanhood. This genesis is marked by regular reproductive cycles and engagement in sexual activity. The gynecologic issues that arise during this period are related to being sexually active. Many young women are emotionally, physically, and mentally vulnerable and this may put them in peril. Being informed about potential gynecologic health risks can empower her to make better informed choices. In addition, some of the problems adolescents face continue to be an issue during this time.

Menstrual-Related Issues

The last time I saw Ingrid, three months ago, she was quite distressed. She had started to experience outbursts of anger, breast tenderness, and abdominal bloating each month. She was worried and somewhat relieved when my examination was found to be unremarkable. I asked her to keep a symptom diary, also noting the onset of her menstruation. She was here to review the diary and gives me a reassuring smile. She had discovered the symptoms occurred approximately 1 week before her period and resolved as soon as her menses started. I then explained that the variation in hormones during a woman's cycle could cause certain symptoms but these are not a sign of anything serious.

Premenstrual Syndrome

Also known as **PMS**, premenstrual syndrome is the cyclic occurrence of symptoms that interfere with the quality of life and is consistently and predictably associated with menses. These symptoms can be physical or emotional in nature. The physical symptoms include breast tenderness, abdominal bloating, headache, and leg swelling. The emotional symptoms include depression, irritability, and outbursts of anger, anxiety, confusion, and social withdrawal.

PMS affects 80 to 85 percent of menstruating women. Most women have mild manifestations and it doesn't interfere with daily functioning. Moderate to severe symptoms occur in 20 to 40 percent of menstruating women, who typically experience 2 to 5 symptoms of **PMS** and report distress associated with these symptoms. More severe symptoms occur in 2 to 10 percent of women.[6] The more severe form is called Premenstrual Dysphoric Disorder.

Physicians typically utilize a symptom diary to make the diagnosis of **PMS** or PMDD. A symptom diary is a record of both emotional and physical symptoms in relationship to the occurrence of menses and should be kept for at least 2 cycles. This record is important in making a diagnosis. PMS symptoms are limited to the part of the cycle that occurs after ovulation, known as the luteal phase. There are some women with other medical problems, such as depressive disorders, migraine headaches, and chronic fatigue syndrome, in which the symptoms are magnified in the luteal phase and can be confused with PMS.

The decision to treat is up to the woman who is experiencing the symptoms. There are no medical consequences to not treating. Managing PMS/PMDD can include medical interventions or behavioral and lifestyle interventions.

Dietary and other lifestyle changes can improve symptoms of PMS. These changes include decreasing the consumption of dairy products, refined sugars, and high-sodium food. Limiting caffeine intake and consuming a low fat and high fiber diet are also recommended. Daily nutritional supplements are also beneficial, especially 400 to 800 mg of magnesium per day, 1200 to 1600 mg of calcium, and 50 to 100 mg of vitamin B6. These supplements have all been proven to alleviate symptoms of PMS. Chasteberry, black cohosh, St. John's wort, ginkgo, and kava may also be beneficial in helping these symptoms. Aerobic exercises, yoga, light therapy, massage therapy, and other relaxation techniques may also be helpful in the mild to moderate cases, especially if used consistently.

Some women elect to use medication to alleviate symptoms. Spironolactone, a diuretic, is helpful in alleviating the bloating that is often a symptom of PMS. Combination hormonal contraceptive pills have been utilized with varying effects and one pill containing drospirenone, a progestin that is like spironolactone has received specific approval for the treatment of PMDD. Menstrual suppression with hormonal methods, such as injectable and implantable progestin hormonal contraceptives and the hormonal IUD, should be effective and are easy to trial on an individual basis. GnRH agonist therapy, such as leuprolide, completely stops ovulation, thereby resolving PMS, but it has limited usefulness because it cannot be used long term.

Serotonin reuptake inhibitors (SRIs) are currently the gold standard for treating PMS and PMDD. They are antidepressants and anxiolytics, meaning they are used primarily to ease anxiety. Drugs in this category include fluoxetine, paroxetine, sertraline, and many others. They can be taken daily or in the 7 to 14 days prior to menses when the symptoms normally occur.

Heavy Bleeding or "Menorrhagia"

Since the delivery of her children, Zena had noticed that her periods have gone from 4 days to 7 days. She changes her pads every hour or two for the first 2 days and can no longer wear a tampon due to the heaviness of the bleeding. She has started to feel more tired and is concerned she might be anemic. "Doc, I'm fed up with having a period. Is there any way you can make it go away?" These are the first words out of her mouth when I enter the examination room. I smile and said "Yes there is, but first let's figure out what's going on."

Menorrhagia is heavy, excessive bleeding with periods or prolonged periods. A typical period last 5 to 7 days with an average blood loss of 80 ml. Bleeding beyond this is a concern for many reasons. First, it is annoying, disruptive, and costly. Pads can be irritating to the skin, and changing sanitary napkins multiple times a day may interfere with productivity. Second, excessive, prolonged bleeding may result in anemia, which could become life-threatening. Finally, the excessive bleeding can be a signal that there is some other problem, such as an unknown pregnancy, a bleeding disorder, a thyroid disorder, or an anatomical abnormality of the uterus such as fibroids or polyps.

An evaluation by a gynecologist is strongly recommended. The assessment will include a thorough history, a physical and pelvic examination, and possibly a laboratory test or other imaging test. Laboratory tests can evaluate thyroid function, measure red blood cell counts to assess levels of anemia, and help determine if there's a bleeding disorder. A pelvic ultrasound is commonly performed to look at the uterus to see if there are any growths, such as fibroids, which can be easily diagnosed. Further studies may be recommended based on the outcome of the above-mentioned tests.

For most women, heavy bleeding can be managed with common medications. Using non-steroidal anti-inflammatory drugs (NSAIDs) such as ibuprofen and naproxen at the onset of the period, and around the clock for the first few days of the period is effective in decreasing the amount of blood loss. For instance, ibuprofen 600 mg every 6 hours for the first 2 days of menstruation can be effective in a woman whose first 2 days of the period are the heaviest. If this isn't effective then hormonal contraception such as the pill, the injection or the hormonal intrauterine device are also extremely effective alternatives. (*See the section on contraception for further details of these medications.*)

Other common problems encountered during this time are irregular or skipped periods, termed "Oligomenorrhea," and painful periods or menstrual cramps, termed "Dysmenorrhea." See Chapter 2 for a detailed discussion of these problems.

Oligomenorrhea can also be related to a thyroid disorder, obesity and insulin resistance or pre-diabetes. It is important to seek medical care to be evaluated for oligomenorrhea because it can be a concern if a woman who experiences it also plans to try to become pregnant in the future. Oligomenorrhea results from anovulation, infrequent ovulation that makes conception difficult or impossible. Medical therapy is available to address this issue.

Dysmenorrhea can be easily treated with NSAIDs, or even hormonal contraception. (*See the section on contraception for details of these medications.*) If the problem persists, further evaluation for other gynecologic problems, like endometriosis, is recommended. (*See the section on pelvic pain in Chapter 4 for a detailed discussion of endometriosis.*)

THE BOTTOM LINE

- PMS, or premenstrual syndrome, affects a large percentage of women.
- Heavy periods or menorrhagia is a common cause of anemia in women and can sometimes lead to hospitalization if left untreated.

- PMS, menorrhagia, and dysmenorrhea can be easily managed with hormonal therapy.

Contraception

During the time when a woman may be sexually active but hasn't yet settled on a life partner and isn't ready to begin a family, she may have multiple concurrent or serial partners. It is important to choose contraception that is effective in preventing both pregnancy and sexually transmitted infections (STIs). Certainly, abstinence is a choice for many, but there are a wide variety of effective methods someone can choose to ensure their health and safety.

I am always so impressed when a young lady comes to my office to discuss contraception before having her first sexual encounter but Nikki earned my deepest admiration. She had decided to become sexually active and wanted to choose a birth control method before her first encounter. She was sure her boyfriend had never had sex before but had insisted that he have all the sexually transmitted infection tests and she had promised to do the same. She also wanted to discuss the options so she could choose the method that was most effective and that would also protect her from infection exposure.

A barrier method like condoms is ideal for preventing sexually transmitted infections if applied appropriately and consistently. The drawbacks are that you have be careful about consistent use and know that there is a risk of the condom tearing or breaking. Hormonal methods are ideal in pregnancy prevention since they are easy to use, effective and have minimal side effects. In addition, a woman doesn't need the cooperation of her male partner. They however do not prevent infections.

The barrier methods work by blocking sperm from getting into the female reproductive tract thus preventing fertilization. The male condom is easily obtained and easy to use. The female condom is also available but not as common or easy to find.

Hormonal methods work in many ways but primarily by preventing the release of an egg from the ovary. If there isn't an egg available to fertilize then pregnancy will not occur. Birth control pills are hormonal contraceptives.

Traditionally, when we refer to birth control pills we mean the estrogen/progestin combination pill. There are currently many pills on the market, their differences typically being variations in the dose and forms of hormone they contain. All pills have the estrogen, also called ethinyl estradiol, but differ by the type of progestin they contain. The dose of estrogen tends to range from 20 to 35 micrograms per pill though a few types contain higher doses. There are many different types of progestins, however, and this tends to distinguish the different brands.

A pill pack typically has 21 active pills, which contain the hormone supplements, and 7 days of inactive pills. These inactive pills do not contain any medication, so it is in this time that menstruation will occur. The different brands may have the same dose of estrogen and progestin in all of the 21 active pills or the dose of the hormones may vary every 7 days.

Contraceptive technology has provided us with newer alternatives for contraceptive delivery. Estrogen/progestin combination contraception can also be delivered by other means. Combination hormonal patches deliver the hormones through the skin. The patch is changed weekly. Leaving the patch off for 7 days on the fourth week then allows a period. There is a contraceptive ring designed for intravaginal delivery. The ring is worn for 3 weeks in a row and removed the fourth week to allow menstruation.

An exciting change in the combination hormonal pill design is that it is available in new formulations that have 24 days of active pills with 4 days of inactive pills. This change decreases even further the side effects and risk of pregnancy.

It is also possible to take the pills in a continuous fashion and have a period when you are ready. There are brands that simplify this process, providing 84 active pills followed by an inactive period of 4 to 7 days, meaning a woman can choose to menstruate only 4 times a year.

The introduction of "the pill" in 1960 gave women the power to control their fertility. This was a historic moment. Over 80 percent of women born after 1945 have used the pill at some point in their lives. The other power this pill provides is the control over menstruation, which is sometimes the primary reason it is used. This is indeed a true medical marvel but it's not perfect.

As with all medications, there are potential risks associated with the pill use, including:

- Thromboembolic events such as heart attacks, stroke, and blood clots in the deep veins and other vessels: This is the major risk and it gradually increases with age.
- Breast cancer (risk only slightly increased)
- Hepatic cancer and noncancerous tumors of the liver (rare)
- Increase in the serum lipids (elevated cholesterol)
- In some women, their age, health status, and habits might contribute to an even higher risk of problems on the pill. The situations in which the pill is not recommended include:
1. Heavy smoking of cigarettes and over age 35: The risk of a thromboembolic event is increased by four-fold compared to a woman over 35 who doesn't smoke.
2. Thromboembolic disorders or a history of a thromboembolic event

3. Severe hypertension
4. Kidney, liver, or adrenal dysfunction
5. Diabetes with vascular involvement
6. Breast cancer
7. Endometrial cancer or other estrogen-dependent cancer
8. Other conditions that might increase the risk of clotting

There are many benefits to taking the birth control pills. They include:

- Effective birth control (>99% effective)
- Regulates menstrual cycle in those with heavy or irregular periods
- Relieves the pain (cramps) that occur with menstruation
- Treats endometriosis
- Prevents recurrent ovarian cyst
- Decreases the risk of ovarian cancer and endometrial cancer
- Treats PMS and PMDD
- Certain types are helpful for acne
- Regulates the onset of menses and decreases the frequency of menstruation

Not everyone tolerates the pill. Side effects or medication intolerance are the major reasons for discontinuation. Common side effects and other pill problems include:

- Spotting and irregular or heavy bleeding
- Nausea/vomiting
- Breast tenderness
- Difficulty remembering to take the pill daily

There is birth control that contains a single hormone: progestin. Progestin-only birth control comes in pill formulations, but is also available as an injectable, as an implant, and as an intrauterine device.

The Essence of You

The lack of estrogen makes this form of birth control attractive to a lot of women.

Progestin-only birth control works in several ways. It suppresses ovulation, the release of the egg from the ovary. If there isn't an egg available, then fertilization can't occur. It also thickens the cervical mucous preventing sperm from traveling through the cervix. If the sperm can't reach the egg, fertilization cannot occur. Finally, it promotes endometrial atrophy by blocking the effects of estrogen on the uterine lining. The lining of the uterus is not prepared for implantation and therefore pregnancy cannot occur.

The advantages of this type of birth control are many. The lack of estrogen means that the risk of problems such as thromboembolic events is much less. Women who are older, smokers, or who have medical problems such as hypertension and diabetes are good candidates for this type of birth control. Progestin-only birth control is also effective in managing heavy bleeding with periods, pain associated with menses, and treating endometriosis.

The progestin-only pill formulation is also referred to as the "mini-pill." The progestin-only pills contain norethindrone, norgestrel, or levonorgesterol—all variations of progestin. This kind of pill must be taken daily because the dose is very low. Thus, the effectiveness for birth control is approximately 93%. However, there isn't a pill-free or inactive pill interval, so it is possible to never have a period while using these pills. This is a popular method in women who are breastfeeding.

The injectable form of progestin is available as Depoprovera. It is a deep intramuscular injection that is given every 12 weeks. It is a high dose progestin, and its effectiveness is greater than 99% due to both the dose level as well as the delivery mechanism. An injection that is given 4 times a year improves compliance. The major drawback to this medication is weight gain. On average women gain 3 to 5 pounds

39

per year while using this medication. Another concern has been the decrease in bone density with long-term use.

This medication can also be delivered via a small implant under the skin of the arm. Implanon is currently available as a single rod-shaped implant that lasts for 3 years. It contains the progestin, etonogestrel, another low-dose formulation. These devices should be removed once they expire.

There are levonorgestrel-containing intrauterine devices (IUDs) that are effective for 3 to 5 years depending on the brand selected. They deliver progestin directly to the endometrial cavity. The serum levels of progestin are much lower in women who use the IUD compared to those who use the pill, implant, or injection. The result is extremely effective birth control with minimal side effects.

The disadvantages of the progestin-only birth control can include irregular, sometimes heavy bleeding, weight gain in some of the methods, and, for certain individuals, an increase in the symptoms of depression. As previously mentioned, there isn't a perfect birth control method. Progestin-only options can provide effective birth control and effective menstrual control with minimal side effects. It is important to partner with your health care provider to choose the method that is right for you.

THE BOTTOM LINE

- Hormonal contraception is the most effective method and the most common choice by young adults.
- Condoms are the only method that will protect against sexually transmitted infections as well as preventing pregnancy.
- Hormonal contraception and condom use in combination are the recommended methods for the prevention of pregnancy and the prevention of sexually transmitted infections.

Sexually Transmitted Infections

I could see that I needed to be extra patient with Penelope, a young college student. She was having a difficult time explaining why she came to see me but it was clear that she was distressed about something. Thankfully it was a slow day and I could spend the time necessary without inconveniencing another patient. I had one of the front office staff bring us some tea and I took her into my office where we sat side by side on the sofa. I chatted about my college experience, asking her a few casual questions along the way. After a few minutes, she opened up. She had recently become sexually active. Against her better judgment, she had intercourse without using a condom with a guy she had just met. Now she was experiencing vaginal irritation, pain with urination and an odorous discharge. She is worried that she may have acquired an infection from that sexual encounter. She had researched providers and found me. "Your patients seem to trust you," she told me.

Sexually transmitted infections are of great concern for women who have become sexually active. Their sexuality is awakening and they are learning what gives them pleasure and what doesn't. Most haven't settled with a life partner, and they may have multiple or serial sexual partners before they do. The risk of exposure to an infection increases with the number of partners and the frequency of unprotected intercourse. The most common types of infections are discussed below.

Chlamydia and **Gonorrhea** are two of the most commonly sexually transmitted infections. They are caused by the bacteria *Chlamydia trachomatis* and *Neisseria gonorrhea,* which can be transmitted through vaginal, anal, and oral intercourse. The bacteria can infect the cervix, urethra, anus, and the throat. In many cases a woman and a man can have the infection and not demonstrate any symptoms. If symptoms are present they may include vaginal discharge, urinary frequency, vaginal irritation or burning, abnormal bleeding, and pain with urination. These infections can be detected with a routine test that can be given at the time of a pelvic examination. Treatment with an antibiotic taken by mouth is generally effective in curing the infections, however all sexual partners must be treated otherwise the risk of reinfection exists.

All sexually active women who are not in a monogamous relationship should be checked routinely for these infections. All young women under the age of 26 should be checked routinely, no matter the status of their relationships. This can be done easily at the time of your annual examination.

If these infections go untreated they can ascend into the uterus and fallopian tubes causing a condition called pelvic inflammatory disease or PID. The symptoms include lower abdominal pain, fever, nausea, and vomiting. It can sometimes be confused with appendicitis. If treatment is not initiated promptly, the risk of developing a life-threatening blood infection is quite high. Sometimes hospitalization is required to control these infections.

Long-term consequences of these infections include infertility, chronic pelvic pain, and ectopic pregnancies. Prevention is the key to avoiding these problems. Always use condoms. Don't have sex with multiple partners or with a partner who has multiple partners. Get tested annually or if you have some concerning symptoms or are suspicious that your partner may be unfaithful.

Herpes is a sexually transmitted infection caused by the virus *Herpes Simplex,* types 1 and 2. It is transmitted during vaginal, anal, and oral intercourse. Typically, it occurs when one partner has active herpes lesions, however the virus can be transmitted when there aren't any apparent sores. A first infection typically occurs 7 to 10 days after exposure with the appearance of painful fluid-filled genital sores that ulcerate. The sores are preceded by fever, fatigue, swollen lymph nodes, and tingling or burning sensations on the genitalia. The sores can be so painful that it causes difficulty with urination, and they can produce a copious discharge. If left untreated the symptoms generally resolve within 2 to 3 weeks, though it can develop into meningitis if a person has a weak immune system. In some cases, the initial outbreak may not be so dramatic.

Herpes infection can be recurrent, meaning some people can experience them more than once. Some people experience frequent recurrences, some infrequent, and others may never experience another outbreak after the first one. The recurrences tend to be shorter and less painful. It is during these outbreaks that the virus can be most easily transmitted to a sexual partner. The virus can also be transmitted to an infant if active lesions are present at the time of vaginal birth and can be potentially life-threatening in a newborn. Thus, it is important that your health care provider is informed of any history of herpes or any other sexually transmitted infection.

Treatment in the form of antiviral oral medication is available to shorten the course of an initial and recurrent infection and to prevent recurrences. The medications are safe and generally well tolerated.

Syphilis is a sexually transmitted infection that people have known about for centuries. It is caused by the bacterial spirochete *Treponema pallidum* and is transmitted sexually even if the transmitting partner is completely asymptomatic, showing no signs of illness.

The initial infection presents with a genital sore called a "chancre," which is the site of entry of the spirochete through the skin. If untreated, the skin lesion resolves in 3 to 6 weeks. The second stage is called secondary syphilis and occurs when the infection gets into the bloodstream. Symptoms include a skin rash, swollen lymph nodes, and fever. This stage lasts for 2 to 6 weeks and also resolves on its own. Then there is a latent phase, when there is no evidence of the infection, during which the organism is still reproducing and transmission of the infection is possible. If untreated, a third of individuals will develop the tertiary stage, which involves infection of the nervous, cardiovascular, and musculoskeletal systems. Meningitis, heart disease, paralysis, and death can result.

If a woman is infected when pregnant, the fetus can become infected too, the consequences of which include fetal death, congenital anomalies, premature delivery, and stillbirth. Again, the key is prevention and early detection. Syphilis infection can be treated with a common antibiotic. A simple blood test can tell a doctor if the patient is infected. The problems in pregnancy and the development of the advanced stages of the infection can be prevented.

Hepatitis B and **Hepatitis C** viral infections are transmitted sexually and through blood transmission, such as a blood transfusion or sharing of needles with illicit drug use. They can also be transmitted to the fetus during pregnancy if the mother is infected. These viruses infect the liver, and while a large percentage of individuals will clear this infection on their own, some will go on to develop chronic hepatitis or liver cirrhosis, and some could die. Liver cancer is another possible consequence. A small percentage of those infected are asymptomatic carriers, meaning they can transmit the infection but don't show any symptoms of the disease. There isn't a specific treatment for hepatitis, but there is a vaccination that is effective for the prevention of Hepatitis B and it is currently a part of routine childhood immunizations. Again, the key is prevention. Using condoms and carefully selecting sexual partners is the key to avoiding all sexually transmitted infections.

HIV is caused by the Human Immunodeficiency Virus. It is transmitted sexually and through blood transmission, like hepatitis. It can easily be transmitted from person to person. This virus infects the blood cells that are important in fighting off infections. Once these immune fighting cells are destroyed the body is without defense and is extremely susceptible to many infections. People who die from

HIV now usually do so because they are undiagnosed and develop a fast-acting infection. Again, the key is prevention, and the use of condoms cannot be overstressed. Further discussion of this infection is beyond the scope of this book, but information on this topic is widely available.

THE BOTTOM LINE

- Your health care provider should be aware of your history of all sexually transmitted infections.
- Sexually transmitted infections have long-term consequences, such as infertility, pelvic pain, and death.
- Abstinence or the use of condoms are the keys to prevention.

HPV and Cervical Dysplasia

"Brianna, why did it take you so long to come back to see me?" I ask firmly. I wanted to scold her for neglecting her health but held my tongue. She had enough to deal with and I needed her to know that I would help get her through this. Last year she had an abnormal pap. I had asked her to return for a special test but she didn't keep the appointment. We had tried to call all her contact numbers but they were disconnected and we didn't receive any response to a registered letter that was sent. Now a year later her pap test is concerning for cervical cancer. She needs to undergo a colposcopy immediately and will likely need surgery.

Cervical cancer is a malignancy of the cervix, known to result from sexual exposure to a virus called Human Papilloma Virus (HPV). Once the cells of the cervix are infected it is possible for the body to fight the infection; however, in some cases the cervix may undergo precancerous changes and eventually develop cancer. This process can happen quickly or it can take 10 or more years. **See Chapter 8 for more details on cervical cancer and its prevention**.

Urinary Tract Infection (UTI)

I had attended Sheila's romantic moonlight wedding just 2 weeks ago. She had married her college sweetheart and they honeymooned in the Virgin Islands. Now she was in my office looking much less than the happy bride. She had started to experience pain with urination, more frequent urination of small amounts of urine, and lower abdominal pain. She was quite relieved when I told her it was probably honeymoon cystitis.

A urinary tract infection or bladder infection occurs when bacteria grow and adhere to the cells lining the bladder. These bacteria typically travel from the vagina and invade the urethra and bladder. Sexual activity is the major factor that tends to increase the risk of an infection. Many young women experience their first UTI shortly after becoming sexually active.

Common symptoms of a urinary tract infection include pain with urination, urinating more frequently, urinating small amounts at a time, and urgency of urination. If left untreated the infection can ascend the urinary tract and to the kidney, at which point it is called pyelonephritis or a kidney infection. The symptoms include abdominal, side, and back pain as well as a fever. Kidney infections are very serious and may require hospitalization for treatment.

An evaluation during routine exams should include a urinalysis and cultures for STIs. A STI can have similar symptoms as a UTI. In some cases, a urine culture to confirm a bacterial infection and to identify the bacteria involved may be required. If a woman has frequent infections other tests may be warranted.

Treatment should include a 3-to-7-day treatment with the appropriate antibiotic for an infection limited to the bladder, and a 10-to-14 day course if involvement of the kidney is suspected.

There are ways to prevent this infection. Drinking plenty of water, wiping from front to back after using the bathroom, urinating after intercourse, and avoiding douching are a few examples. Acidifying your urine by drinking cranberry juice or taking cranberry tablets is helpful.

THE BOTTOM LINE

- Urinary tract infections (UTIs) are common in sexually active women.
- If untreated, an infection could ascend to the kidneys causing a more serious infection that might require hospitalization.
- If a UTI occurs more than 2 to 3 times a year it is considered recurrent and you should see your health care provider to discuss measures to minimize these recurrences.

Chapter 4

The Reproductive Years: The Advent

The advent of this period comes with gynecologic needs related to reproduction or being sexually active. Sexually transmitted infections, vaginitis, and problems with the gynecologic organs are more frequent during this phase of life. This chapter will review some of the common problems women face during this time.

Vaginitis

I see Deidre, my hairstylist, at least twice a month. She keeps my hair healthy and looking fashionable. Over the past few months she has been constantly complaining about vaginal discharge and odor. Despite multiple visits to her doctor, it keeps coming back. I finally say, "Deidre, why don't you come see me?" "Listen doc," she replies, I respect you and all but I don't think I can face you after you've had a look my privates." "Get over it girl," I reply. "Come see me. Let's fix this problem and then you and I can pretend that I never saw that part of you. As a matter of fact, I've examined so many women I wouldn't remember anyway." She laughed and finally agreed to come to my office for an exam.

Vaginal discharge, odor, and irritation are the "bane of the female existence". It is by far the most common reason for a gynecologic visit. The symptoms cause a great deal of annoyance, distress, discomfort, and seemingly occur at the most inconvenient time.

Most women worry that these symptoms indicate a serious problem or that their partner has been unfaithful. The irritation and discomfort can be distracting, taking priority over other important concerns. The irresistible urge to scratch and embarrassing odor can create such distress that for most women solving the problem becomes the primary goal for the day.

Unfortunately for most women, gynecologists don't necessarily view it as an emergency, or even an urgent problem, so getting in to see a health care provider can sometimes be a challenge. This section will describe the common causes of vaginitis and how they are typically managed in the hope that it will bring some reassurance, guidance, and relief to those who suffer from it.

Vaginitis is an inflammation of the vagina, and the cause can be infectious or noninfectious. In many cases the vulva, the area that includes the external anatomy, is also affected. The symptoms can be varied but usually include one or more of the following: an unusual discharge, itching, irritation, swelling, discomfort, pain, odor, and pain with intercourse. These symptoms are common in a lot of gynecological problems, including sexually transmitted infections, but the most likely cause is *Candida* vaginitis (vaginal yeast), bacterial vaginosis, or trichomoniasis.

Candida or Yeast

A yeast or candida infection—also referred to as "thrush"—occurs when the normal flora, or "good bacteria", of the vaginal tract are disrupted, leading to an overgrowth of the candida fungus. The symptoms are often distracting and distressing, and they can interfere with a woman's daily activities and decrease the quality of her relationships or even work productivity. Immediate treatment is required so she can get back to normal life.

Candida organisms are a normal part of the vaginal flora, detectable in up to 50 percent of women. Between 40 and 75 percent of women will experience a yeast infection in their lifetimes[1]. It isn't a problem until there is an overgrowth, leading to symptoms like itching, burning, and vaginal odor. Fortunately, it is also usually easy to treat, though approximately 5 percent of women experience chronic or recurrent problems that can be frustrating and expensive.

Typical symptoms include vulvar itching, burning, pain, and stinging during urination. The examining physician may find redness, swelling, fissures (skin cracks), and a thick, curd-like discharge. Even though the symptoms are usually enough to make a diagnosis, it is important to have objective testing as other infections are found as much as 72 percent of the time.

Testing methods include a potassium hydroxide (**KOH**) prep, gram stain, or culture. The **KOH** prep can be done by a doctor on the spot. A sample of the discharge and a couple of drops of **KOH** are placed on a slide and examined under a microscope to look for the presence of candida. Gram stains and cultures must be sent to a lab for determination. The gram stain results are usually available within a couple of days while the culture may take several. The **KOH** and the gram stain tests provide quick results, allowing for immediate treatment, while the culture is much more accurate and may identify cases missed by the other tests.

The culture is especially important in cases of recurrence or chronic infections because it can identify the specific organism involved. Although the majority of infections are due to *candida albicans*, other types, such as *candida tropicalis,* can be the culprit in up to 23 percent of cases[2]. This is important to know because the response to treatment may be variable and different types of candida can be resistant to commonly used antifungals.

Treatment is usually delivered vaginally with either a cream or suppository, and can require 1-, 3-, or 7-day therapies. The shorter courses tend to have more concentrated medication whose treatment effects last several days. This more concentrated form, however, can lead to genital irritation. The most commonly available medications include clotrimazole, miconazole, butoconazole, tioconazole and terconazole. The first four are available over the counter without a prescription. Fluconazole is available for oral use but a prescription is required in many countries.

Candida infections tend to occur more often in the second half of a woman's cycle, in the setting of condom use, and in those who have intercourse more than four times per month. Other risk factors include young age, recent antibiotic use, and other concurrent infections. It is unclear why some women develop frequent recurrent infections, though they often have a higher rate of vaginal colonization with candida.

Women with frequent recurrent infections can be given chronic courses of antifungal medication in an attempt to suppress the infections. This can be done with weekly local or oral therapy for 3 to 6 months. There isn't any clear way of preventing these infections, but I have had patients who controlled the problem by limiting their intake of simple carbohydrates and other foods that support candida.

Even though this problem is the source of great distress, it isn't life threatening and many options exist for managing the infections. The drugs mentioned above are generic names, so be aware that many are marketed under different brand names and that you may have to ask the pharmacist for help when you are making a purchase. It is important to seek consultation with a health care provider if you are experiencing problems with recurrence or if you are not responding to the over-the-counter treatments.

Denise Howard, MD

Bacterial Vaginosis

This is the most common cause of non-transmissible genital tract infections in women. Bacterial vaginosis results from an overgrowth of a specific bacterium. When the flora of the genital tract is disrupted, one bacterial type may overgrow, producing a discharge and an awful odor. In usual circumstances this does not cause any long-term harm, but most women desire treatment because the symptoms are annoying.

There is a microcosm of organisms in the genital tract that maintains a perfect balance; sometimes this is disrupted causing numerous problems. The predominant bacteria there are the *lactobacilli*, which produce substances that keep the tissue at a low, acidic pH, protecting against potentially harmful organisms. When the *lactobacilli* are destroyed, the environment is more susceptible to new infection as well as vulnerable to specific bacterial overgrowth.

Bacterial infection, bacterial vaginosis, gardnerella or nonspecific vaginitis are the common terms used to describe the condition. Organisms that have been identified as the culprit in these infections include: *Gardnerella, Bacteroides, Mobiluncus, Peptococcus, Eubacterium* and *Mycoplasma*. No matter which bacteria are found on culture, the clinical findings are the same; a copious grayish-white discharge with the consistency of milk and a foul odor. Many women also report that the odor is worse after intercourse.

It appears that there are multiple causes of this infection. Many studies have identified factors that make a woman more likely to develop bacterial vaginosis, including douching, smoking, pregnancy, and having intercourse at the time of menstruation. The association with douching has been confirmed in many studies.

On examination, the physician will see the typical discharge as described above. A confirmatory diagnosis is based on a combination of findings. These include a pH greater than 4.5, a fishy or amine-like odor when 10 percent potassium hydroxide (KOH) is added to a sample of the discharge, clue cells seen under the microscope, absence of *lactobacilli* and a culture showing the predominant growth of one of the bacteria mentioned above. Clue cells are epithelial cells that are studded with *coccobacilli* and have a classic appearance on microscopic examination, making it easy for a healthcare provider to make the diagnosis in the office.

The standard treatment has been oral metronidazole 500 mg twice daily for 7 days. This is effective in about 96 percent of cases. Some women experience gastrointestinal upset and a metallic taste after taking the medication. In addition, it should not be taken within 12 hours of consuming alcohol because it can amplify the alcohol effect, leading to severe "hangover" symptoms. An alternative is clindamycin 300 mg orally twice daily for 7 days, which has about a 94 percent success rate. The drawback is that it can cause diarrhea in a small percentage of women.

Local therapies in the form of ovules—small, bullet-shaped pellets that are inserted directly in the vagina—creams and gels have been developed to avoid some of the side effects mentioned above. This provides a safer treatment option for pregnant women. These medications include clindamycin ovules 100 mg for 3 nights, clindamycin 2 percent cream nightly for 7 nights, and metronidazole gel twice daily for 5 days.

Tinidazole is a new oral medication that can be given as 1 gram daily for 5 days or 2 grams daily for 2 days. This shorter treatment period is appealing and the characteristics of the drug make it likely to be equally effective as the older therapies.

Bacterial vaginosis has been associated with preterm labor, postpartum uterine infections, and pelvic infections after hysterectomy. Thus, it is important to be treated and to control recurrent infections. If you have any of the risk factors listed above, you should seek treatment if you develop any of the symptoms described in this section. In addition, some of the risk factors can be eliminated, and it is within your power to make changes that may improve your health.

Trichomoniasis

Trichomoniasis, also called trich, is the most common non-viral sexually transmitted infection in the U.S. It is also the third most common cause of vaginitis and, like the other two, does not cause any long-term harm if treated quickly and completely. As with the other causes of vaginitis, the symptoms tend to drive women to seek care, but this pathogen is more insidious and resilient, making complete eradication challenging.

The causative organism is *Trichomonas Vaginalis*, a protozoan parasite whose only host is human. It resides in the lower genital tract of both men and women, including the urethra, and is efficiently transmitted during intercourse. It is able to survive for hours in excreted urine or semen and on soiled towels or underwear used by infected women. Thus non-sexual transmission is possible but not likely.

Typical symptoms include a copious odorous vaginal discharge that may have a range in colors, like clear, white, grey and green. Other symptoms may include itching, pain with urination, frequent urination, urgent urination, pain with intercourse, and lower abdominal discomfort. It can take a few days to several weeks to develop symptoms after exposure and over 50 percent of people never develop any symptoms[3]. This contributes to continued transmission and even chronic infestation lasting years, even decades.

Many women come to their doctors complaining of symptoms that may lead to detection. Some doctors perform routine checks for these types of infections because they recognize that they can be present without causing problems. Even though trichomoniasis does not generally cause direct harm, detecting and treating it is wise. It can increase the rate of HIV transmission in exposed women and it has been associated with preterm labor, premature rupture of membranes and low birth weight infants in women who are infected during pregnancy.

The diagnosis can be made easily with several readily available tests. A wet mount is the oldest, more readily available method. It consists of taking a small sample of vaginal secretion and placing in a drop of saline solution on a slide with cover. Microscopic examination can easily identify the protozoa under ideal situations. An ovoid-shaped organism with a flagellated structure can be seen swimming amongst epithelial and white blood cells. These protozoa with their amoeboid-like movements have a classic appearance on microscopic examination, but can be missed if the number of organisms is low or if their motility is decreased.

Other methods for detecting trichomonas include rapid point of care tests and culture. The point of care test utilizes methods that detect genetic material or specific structural markers of the organism. These tests have a high sensitivity and can be completed in 10 to 45 minutes. Cultures may take up to a week, but combined with the wet mount can yield a nearly 100 percent detection rate.

Treatment consists of an oral medication that is also used to treat other bacterial and parasitic infections. Metronidazole 2 grams as a single dose or tinidazole 2 grams, also as a single dose, is the standard therapy. If sexual partners are not treated at the same time, there is a high chance of recurrence. Reinfection rates of up to 17 percent have been reported. There are also reports of low-level resistance to the medication. In these scenarios treatment consists of metronidazole 500 mg twice daily for 7 days or either of the above medications at a dose of 2 grams daily for 5 days.

Because of the theoretical risk of birth defects, treatment in pregnant women should be delayed until after the first trimester is completed. If a pregnant woman has symptoms, local or intravaginal treatment with clotrimazole is an alternative. It is important, however, to treat her as soon as possible and recheck to ensure the treatment has been effective to prevent pregnancy complications.

THE BOTTOM LINE

- Some vaginal discharge is normal. Odor, itching, and irritation are signs that there is something wrong.
- Over-the-counter anti-fungals, such as miconazole, only work for candida (yeast infections).
- If your symptoms are recurrent, you need to see a gynecologist to make sure you don't have a sexually transmitted infection.
- Some women have recurrent vaginitis and need to be treated with a specific regimen to prevent recurrence.

Uterine Fibroids

I've taken care of Shareena for a long time. She's had fibroids since age 25. I removed most of them for her at age 27 and then performed 3 cesarean sections to deliver her four healthy children, including one set of twins. I performed a tubal ligation the last time and was happy about it because the surgery was extremely difficult and Shareena lost a lot of blood. I thought I wouldn't have to go back in but now she is back with heavy bleeding, severe anemia and a fibroid uterus the size of a term pregnancy. "Take it all out doc. I'm over this," she shouts as she takes a seat in my office after I had a chance to examine her and review her blood test results.

What are fibroids?

Fibroids, or leiomyoma, are another of the most common reasons women seek care from a gynecologist. They account for 70 to 80 percent of all benign tumors of the female genital tract[9]. But what are they? Fibroids are tumors made of smooth muscle. The other term used to describe this tumor is "leiomyoma." They can occur anywhere in the body, but the uterus is the most common site. They can develop unnoticed or cause life-threatening problems; however, the tumors themselves typically are not cancerous.

The uterus is the pear-shaped organ located within the pelvis organ that can support the growth of a fetus. The upper portion has two branching areas called the fallopian tubes, which terminate at the ovaries. The lower portion of the uterus terminates into the cervix, which is the opening to the uterine cavity and the structure that dilates during childbirth. The surface of the uterus, called the serosa, is lined with peritoneal tissue. The major portion of the uterus is a smooth muscle layer, which contracts to expel menstrual tissue or the fetus. The endometrium is the lining of the uterus, which is a vascular rich area that supports the developing fetus, and which women shed during their menstruation.

Fibroids are found in various sites of the uterus. Fibroids growing in the lining of the uterus are described as "submucosal" because they are beneath the mucosal layer (the endometrium). If they are located within the muscle of the uterus the term "intramural" is used. Subserosal fibroids are located on the surface of the uterus. Subserosal fibroids can sometimes grow like a flower grows on a stalk, in which case it is "pedunculated." Sometimes these pedunculated fibroids can become parasitic, attaching to the intestine and developing a means to a regular blood supply. In unusual cases the fibroids can grow in the broad ligaments, which are the supportive and connecting structures that attach the reproductive organ to the abdominal sidewalls and through which the vasculature travels.

Fibroids can range in size from 1 cm up to 15 cm or more. A woman's uterus can contain 1 or multiple tumors. These fibroids can grow in a variety of locations, creating serious problems for the woman. It isn't unusual for fibroids to increase the size of the uterus to that of a term pregnancy or even larger.

The chance of a woman having fibroids increases with age. The reported prevalence is approximately 15 percent in women but up to 50 percent in premenopausal women and more than 70 percent of women over the age of 50 [10, 11]. There appears to be some genetic connection in that the problem is more prevalent in family members of women with fibroids. The condition is even more prevalent in certain ethnic groups—the highest in those of African origin. Black women are 3 times more likely to have uterine fibroids compared to white women.

This prevalent benign tumor can cause significant problems for reproductive-age women. Women who have never had children are also at greater risk of developing fibroids. If left un-treated they can cause life-threatening problems or decrease fertility. Many treatment options are available for managing these tumors.

Problems Caused by Fibroids

Fibroids are the most common tumor of the female genital tract. If a woman has a growth in the pelvic region it is most likely a fibroid. Up to two-thirds of women suffer from this condition. A woman can have fibroids for many years before they are detected. They can sometimes be found during a routine pelvic exam, or a woman might experience problems caused by the fibroids.

Some of these problems include irregular or heavy periods—the most common problem that women with fibroids experience. Sometimes these can be so severe, especially in cases of intramural fibroids, that a woman may develop anemia and need a blood transfusion. Women describe passing large clots and needing to change their pads or tampons as often as every hour, or even less. They typically experience a set number of heavy days, and the menstruation might last up to 10 days. Women who have a submucosal fibroid usually complain of bleeding or spotting between periods, but some experience bleeding that just doesn't seem to stop.

A woman may also develop increasing abdominal size which can cause constipation, urinary frequency, and pelvic pressure and pain. A pedunculated fibroid can move and contribute to intermittent pressure symptoms like difficulty urinating or defecating. Another hallmark of uterine fibroids is severe pain with menstrual bleeding. Depending on their location, fibroids can cause problems with infertility, preterm labor, and growth restriction in a developing pregnancy. As fibroids enlarge, the blood supply that they receive from the uterine vessels may be dramatically decreased. The fibroid can attach to other pelvic organs, such as the bowels, and develop a new blood supply. When this occurs, it is described as being "parasitic." If it is unable to obtain an additional blood supply, the tissues can die, causing severe pain and fever. This process is called "degeneration."

Typically, fibroid symptoms develop gradually and may remain unnoticed for some time. Routine gynecologic examinations are recommended. The gynecologist's suspicions might be raised based on the description of blood loss with menstruation, or she might feel a mass on pelvic examination. Sometimes significant anemia is revealed on a routine blood count, which would then lead to further testing.

All women are at risk of developing fibroids. If you experience any of the above symptoms, it is important to discuss them with your doctor. There isn't any reason to be frightened because this condition rarely develops into cancer, but it is important to seek early treatment as it can affect fertility or cause significant inconvenience.

What causes fibroids?

The etiology of these tumors is currently being studied and there are many potential contributors to the development of fibroids. Because this problem is limited to reproductive-aged women, hormones must play a role. One theory suggests that the hormones have a strong effect on local growth factors, inciting excessive growth in certain smooth muscle cells.

Recent advances in genetic research have allowed better understanding of these tumors. The fact that they are more common in first-degree relatives of women with fibroids and that the prevalence is much higher in black women suggest a genetic cause.

All the cells in our body typically have the same chromosomes. Sometimes cells can become damaged, causing the chromosomes inside it to become abnormal. Studies of fibroids have shown that 60 percent of the cells have normal chromosomes and 40 percent have abnormal chromosomes.[6] When the abnormal chromosomes are examined in greater detail, certain patterns of gene abnormalities are found, suggesting there are numerous different gene abnormalities that lead to fibroid tumors.

Why is this relevant? There is an association between the sizes of the tumors and their chromosomal make up—their "karyotype." There is also an association between recurrence of fibroids and the karyotype of the tumors. Looking at a tumor's genetic makeup may also be helpful in predicting which of these tumors will develop into cancer.

Finally, there is a rare but life-threatening syndrome called hereditary leiomyomatosis and renal cell carcinoma. Affected individuals will have smooth muscle tumors that form under their skin (cutaneous), uterine fibroids, and an increased risk of malignant tumors. The malignancy presents in the kidney (renal cell carcinoma), meaning that there are large tumors in the kidney that have usually spread (metastasized) by the time the cancer is diagnosed. These women are also at high risk of leiomyosarcoma, which is a malignant fibroid tumor. These malignancies occur as a part of this syndrome and tend to affect younger women. Thus, it is important to know your family medical history and report it to your gynecologist if there's a family history of cutaneous fibroids, malignant fibroids, and kidney cancer.

The Evaluation

The most common tool used to evaluate for fibroids is the pelvic ultrasound, which can be done trans-abdominally and trans-vaginally and during which the uterus and ovaries are easily visualized. The size of the uterus is measured and individual fibroids can be counted and measured. If more detailed visualization of the lining of the uterus is required, a saline injection ultrasound or hysterosonogram can be performed. A saline solution is instilled into the uterine lining through the cervix. Ultrasound scanning can then image the lining in detail. This is the easiest way to determine if there are submucosal fibroids or endometrial polyps.

The density of the abdominal wall or the size and bulkiness of the fibroid can sometimes limit ultrasound imaging. In these cases, magnetic resonance imaging (MRI) can give an even more detailed picture of the uterus, fibroids, their location and size. It is more expensive than ultrasound and its use should be reserved for select circumstances.

A hysteroscopy is an alternative procedure to the hysterosonogram that allows direct visualization of the lining of the uterus. Submucosal fibroids, endometrial polyps, and other endometrial abnormalities can be easily visualized by the surgeon and potentially treated at the same time via resection or vaporization.

The above diagnostic tools are commonly used to assess uterine fibroids. The information obtained during these procedures can help your gynecologist recommend treatment options that are appropriate for your individual circumstance. Fibroids are not always the cause of the problem and they don't always need to be removed. Your physician should partner with you to select the least invasive and most effective option to address your problem.

Medical Treatment

Just because fibroids are present doesn't mean that they need to be removed. In many cases, they are present, but don't cause any problems so should be left alone. Sometimes the problems that are thought to be due to fibroids can be controlled without surgery. There are many medical options available.

Non-steroidal anti-inflammatory drugs such as ibuprofen reduce prostaglandin release in the uterus, decreasing the pain associated with menstruation but also decreasing the blood loss by about 30 percent. To minimize gastrointestinal side effects, their use should be limited to 5 days.

Anti-fibrinolytic drugs have been proven to be helpful with menstrual blood loss, even when caused by fibroids. Tranexamic acid has been approved by the Food and Drug Administration for the treatment of heavy periods. Other agents are available in other countries. However, women who are at increased risk of venous thromboembolism should avoid this medication.

Heavy bleeding with periods and painful periods can sometimes be controlled with hormones such as those used in hormonal contraception. Birth control regimens can result in shorter and less-painful periods. There are many brands and dosing regimens, available as pills, patches, injections, and transvaginal rings. They can be used cyclically or continuously. There is also an intrauterine device and a cutaneous implant that delivers hormones. These provide coverage for 2 to 5 years. It is important to work with your doctor to identify the regimen that works for you. You should try them for at least 3 months to determine their effectiveness.

Other medical treatments include injectable therapies that trick the brain into thinking that you are in menopause. These are called GnRH agonist or antagonists. Goserelin, leuprolide, and nafarelin are commonly used. If the ovary is temporally dormant, it does not produce hormones and the fibroids gradually shrink. This can allow for temporary bleeding control, making other surgical therapies more effective. The absence of menses also allows time for the body to resolve the anemia. The most common side effect of this form of therapy is hot flashes. Once the medication is stopped, the fibroids typically return to their pretreatment size unless a woman is close to menopause.

Mifepristone, a progesterone receptor modulator, taken in a daily dose of 5 to 50 mg a day has been shown to shrink fibroids when used over a 3 to 6-month period. It works by blocking the progesterone receptors in the uterus. Thus, the uterus and fibroids shrink. Clinical studies demonstrate a reduction in the fibroid volume of 26 to 74 percent. Potential concerns are the development of endometrial hyperplasia and liver effects in a small percentage of women. Other selective progesterone receptor modulators and anti-progestins are being studied and hopefully will provide an even broader array of options for the treatment of fibroids.

Surgical Management

Not every woman with fibroids will require treatment, but those who do may not be able to manage them with medical therapy. Surgical therapy and procedures are available to manage the problems if medical treatments fail.

Uterine fibroid embolization is an alternative for women who desire a minimally invasive option for managing their fibroids. The procedure entails injecting synthetic particles in the artery feeding the uterus to obstruct the vessels. The result is a decrease in the blood supply to the fibroids and they shrink over time. It is very effective in reducing the amount of blood loss with periods and in decreasing the bulk of the uterus. Some women don't have periods after this procedure. Approximately 80 percent of women have improvement in their symptoms and 91 percent of those undergoing the procedure report satisfaction with the therapy.[12]

There are potential but rare complications of the procedure. The most common, of course, is failure. A small percentage of women undergo premature menopause due to problems with their ovarian blood supply. There are also rare reported cases of embolization of unintended vessels (blockages preventing blood flow) compromising blood supply to other tissue.

A new technique utilizes **MRI** to guide focused ultrasound beams through the anterior abdominal wall and into the fibroid. This results in thermal ablation of the treated fibroid. This procedure allows for precise targeting of the fibroid and significant improvement in the symptoms.

If you desire to retain your fertility potential, it is best to consider a surgical procedure called a myomectomy. After a surgical incision, the individual fibroids are removed and the uterus repaired with sutures. This typically results in a normal-sized uterus. Selective skilled surgeons can also perform this procedure via laparoscopy, which has become more widely available after improvements in laparoscopic techniques and tools. For some women, this can be a permanent fix; others may experience a recurrence over time.

Hysterectomy is an alternative for women who have completed their childbearing and want a definitive treatment. If the uterus is removed there is no chance for recurrence of the fibroids. Removing the uterus does not result in menopause; only removing the ovaries will bring on menopause. A hysterectomy can be performed vaginally, abdominally, or laparoscopically with or without robotic assistance. The surgical route is dependent on a number of factors, but the most important include the size of the uterus, the skill set of the surgeon, and the availability of necessary resources to facilitate the procedure.

There are several available procedures that can treat uterine fibroids. It is important for you to seek the care of an experienced gynecologist who can provide you with a comprehensive evaluation and counsel you on the options that best meet your needs.

THE BOTTOM LINE

- Leiomyoma (fibroids) are a common problem and treatment is only needed if they are causing problems.
- There are many options for addressing the problems caused by fibroids.
- Surgery may be required but it shouldn't be the first treatment choice. Seek a second opinion if you are not satisfied with the options provided by your doctor.

Pelvic Pain

Margaret has come to see me for an umpteenth opinion, as she so aptly describes it. She is highly frustrated. "Doctor, I need your honest opinion. I have seen so many doctors and each has a different opinion about what I have. I'm frustrated and all I know is I need someone to fix this pain," she declared as she dumped a pile of medical papers on my desk. "I have been told that I have endometriosis, interstitial cystitis, ovarian cysts, and other things I can't even pronounce. Please help me."

Pelvic pain is a common complaint in women. A gynecologic cause is often assumed but it is important to remember that there are other organs that reside in the pelvis. It is perfectly acceptable to start the evaluation process with a primary care physician or a gynecologist, but if the problem persists further evaluation by another specialist may be required.

When communicating with your provider, it is important to be clear and concise. They will be interested in the timing of the pain. How long has the pain been present? Is it constant or intermittent? Note the location of the pain and if it radiates. Describe the pain. Is it sharp, dull, cramping, or burning? Grade the severity of the pain. Is it mild, moderate, or severe? What brings on the pain and what appears to ease it? What is the relationship of the pain to menstruation?

The health care provider may also ask questions about urinary symptoms, gastrointestinal symptoms, vaginal irritation or discharge, and sexual habits. Urinary frequency, pain with urination, and urinary urgency suggest a urinary source for the pain, such as a urinary tract infection. Nausea, vomiting, and poor appetite suggest a gastrointestinal source, such as appendicitis. Vaginal discharge and a new sexual partner are suggestive of a gynecologic infection as the source.

A physical examination, including a pelvic examination, should be performed. A rectal examination may also be necessary. Your doctor may require cervical cultures, urine cultures, and blood work. Other diagnostic tests might include a CT scan, pelvic ultrasound, or other imaging test, as well as a colonoscopy or a diagnostic laparoscopy.

Pelvic pain could be caused by many gynecologic, urologic, or gastrointestinal issues. It is important to know that physicians are anxious to eliminate cancer as the possible source of the pain, but this is a rare cause. Urologic causes include urinary tract infections, kidney stones, and interstitial cystitis. Gastrointestinal causes may include appendicitis, constipation, irritable bowel syndrome, diverticulitis, and colon cancer. Gynecologic causes include pelvic inflammatory disease, ovarian cyst, ovulation, fibroids, endometriosis, ovarian torsion, ectopic pregnancy, and malignancy. It is important to know that pelvic pain may also result from musculoskeletal or myofascial causes.

Pain management is dependent on both the presenting symptoms and the test results. If the pain is chronic in nature, resolution may take some time. It is important to be cooperative and patient in the evaluation. The following sections review common gynecologic causes of pelvic pain.

What is endometriosis?

Endometriosis is the most common cause of chronic pelvic pain in women. It occurs in approximately 10 percent of menstruating women, 38 percent of infertile women and is found in close to 80 percent of women who have chronic pain. The pain can sometimes be quite debilitating, interfering with the quality of life.[13]

It is a chronic, relapsing condition with an unknown trigger. There appears to be a slight genetic association as there is a 7 to 10 percent increase of risk in women with an affected first-degree relative and a strong concordance in identical twins. Other risk factors include never pregnant, onset of menarche before age 11, cycles less than 27 days and heavy prolonged menses. Women, who have delivered more children, had a longer period of breast-feeding and exercise more than 4 hours per week are less likely to develop endometriosis. The course is unpredictable for the individual but of those with a known diagnosis, 29 percent will worsen, 42 percent will have persistent but unchanged symptoms and 29 percent will experience improvement over time without treatment. Even those who are treated have a 45 percent chance of recurrence after 5 years.[14]

Endometriosis is the implantation of endometrial tissue in sites other than the uterus. Endometriotic implants are commonly found in the pelvic cavity, growing on the ovaries and tubes, and in the peritoneum behind the uterus, over the bladder, on the abdominal sidewall, and over the rectum. Less common sites include abdominal incisions, in the bladder, and in the wall of the rectum. There are even reported cases of it being found in the lungs.

No one knows how endometrial tissue gets to these sites but there are a few theories. One theory is that of retrograde menstruation, meaning that the endometrium, which is normally shed through the cervix and out of the body through the vagina, is shed back through the fallopian tube and into the pelvis. This tissue then implants and grows in response to estrogen. It is common to find menstrual blood in the pelvis during menstruation if a laparoscopy is performed at the time of menses.

Another theory is that the tissue in the pelvis undergoes a transformation called metaplasia, changing into endometrial tissue that then responds to hormonal fluctuation. The last theory involves the metastasis of the endometrial tissue. The tissue travels from the uterus via the blood stream or lymphatic system to the affected sites, implanting and growing in response to estrogen.

The ectopic endometrial tissue grows and changes in response to increased estrogen levels, which also fluctuate through the ovulatory cycle. These are the same changes the endometrium goes through to prepare for the implantation of a fertilized egg and to shed if implantation does not occur. Thus, the pain of endometriosis is typically cyclic, especially in the early stages. The presence of the tissue in the pelvis causes adhesion formation and scarring, which also contributes to the pain. Sometimes the tissue can grow on the ovary, producing a cyst called an endometrioma.

Not every woman who has endometriosis will experience pain, but for those who do the pain can be progressive. Pain with the period, premenstrual pain, and infertility are the most common indicators of this condition. In some cases, the pain can be managed with analgesics or hormonal therapy, but a definitive diagnosis can only be made by surgery.

<u>Diagnosing Endometriosis</u>

Initially, a woman may experience painful cramps with her period. Gradually this becomes severe and then starts to occur 1 to 2 days before the period. Eventually this time frame may extend to 1 to 2 weeks before the period. Many women report only being pain-free the week after their period. The pain can range from mild to severe, and for some this pain can be quite debilitating.

The daily pain is usually worse with the onset of the period. It is typically described as a lower abdominal cramping. Some women complain of back pain as well, or pain that can radiate into the thighs. The pain that occurs outside of the period can be intermittent and sharp or constant. Other symptoms may include pain with intercourse during deep thrusting as well as urinary and bowel complaints. Some women may experience the pain for years before a diagnosis is made.

There are other causes of pelvic pain that may present in a similar fashion. Chronic interstitial cystitis may present with pain that is worse during the period, and some women suffer from both conditions.

Women can also experience pain with intercourse that may be due to pelvic adhesions or a pelvic mass. Irritable bowel syndrome is another cause of pelvic pain that may be confused with endometriosis.

Some women who have endometriosis do not experience pain. They may come to their doctor's office seeking help with infertility and endometriosis is found during the evaluation process. It may also be an incidental finding at the time of surgery for some other issue, such as a tubal ligation. Sometimes a pelvic mass is noted on routine examination that is later found to be an endometrioma.

Treatment can be initiated based on symptoms. It is important, however, to evaluate for other potential causes of pain. A pelvic examination, cultures, and ultrasound can detect other causes of pain. A definitive diagnosis of endometriosis can only be made from looking inside the pelvis. A laparoscopy is the most common route. Endometriosis has a typical appearance, but sometimes the appearance may not be classic. A biopsy for histopathological evaluation is often recommended to confirm the diagnosis. Once a diagnosis is made, appropriate treatment can be initiated.

Medical Treatment of Endometriosis

The initial presentation of endometriosis is typically pain with the onset of menses. This is called dysmenorrhea. Nonsteroidal anti-inflammatory drugs can be effective in relieving this pain. Taking the medication as prescribed, around-the-clock for the most painful days of the period, can significantly reduce the pain. Initiating this medication 1 to 2 days before the onset of the period can also be effective in preventing the pain from occurring. This typically means 600 mg of ibuprofen every 6 hours or 800 mg every 8 hours and 550 mg of naproxen every 12 hours. It is important to limit the use of these drugs to only a few days because they can cause gastritis (irritated stomach lining) or stomach ulcers. Women with an allergy to aspirin should avoid this medication and those who have asthma should consult their health care provider before using it.

The next treatment tier for pelvic pain due to endometriosis is the use of hormones. Birth control pills used in the traditional manner have a very high chance of relieving the pain. Initially it can be combined with drugs such as ibuprofen; some women find that they may no longer need this drug after being on the pill for 3 months or more. Birth control pills can be used in a continuous fashion to address the pain associated with menstruation. Standard birth control pills can be manipulated so that menses occur 3 to 4 times a year or not at all. Other hormones that are also effective in treating the pain of endometriosis include progestin-only methods. These methods are described in detail in the section on contraception.

Medications Used for Severe Endometriosis

If standard medical management isn't effective, your gynecologist may suggest more aggressive measures. Gonadotropin releasing hormone (GnRH) agonists are one of the most commonly used medications in the treatment of severe or persistent endometriosis. They are similar to the gonadotropin-releasing hormone produced in the brain that tells the pituitary gland to release FSH and LH, which in turn tells the ovaries to ovulate. GnRH agonists binds to the GnRH receptors changing the message delivered to the pituitary gland. The release of eggs from the ovary is temporarily suspended and estrogen production drops, then the endometriosis shrinks. This treatment is typically used for 6 months but can be used longer under select circumstances.

There are 3 widely available GnRH agonists. Leuprolide (Lupron) is an intramuscular injection, which can be given as a monthly or every-twelfth-week injections. Goserelin (Zoladex) is given as a subcutaneous implant, which also is prescribed monthly or every 12 weeks. Nafarelin (Synarel) is given as a twice daily nasal spray. These medications produce a medical menopause, which lasts as long as the medication is prescribed. In menopause, a woman's estrogen levels are extremely low and the endometriotic implants resolve due to a lack of estrogen. The most common side effects include hot flashes, night sweats, urogenital atrophy, bone loss, and sleep disturbance. Most of these symptoms can be managed with add-back therapy. Treatment results in an 85 percent reduction in pelvic pain, pain with intercourse, and menstrual pain.

An older and now less-widely used treatment is Danazol. It has a progestin-like effect and has been shown to reduce mild to moderate endometriosis related pain by 80 percent at 2 months. The dose is 400 to 800 mg daily. The androgenic side effects of acne, facial hair, decreased breast density, and other masculinizing symptoms makes it much less popular than other treatments.

The development of aromatase inhibitors has provided an additional tool in the treatment of hormonally related problems. Two of the most common aromatase inhibitors are Anastrozole, 1 mg daily and Letrozole, 2.5 mg daily. These medications work by blocking the production of estrogen, thus creating a menopause-like state. The side effects are therefore similar to the GnRH agonists.

Surgical Treatment of Endometriosis

If medical therapy for endometriosis is no longer effective, surgical options exist to address this problem. Surgery can be both diagnostic and therapeutic. A laparoscopy to diagnose endometriosis typically is the next step in the treatment process if pelvic pain has not responded to standard medication. This procedure is done under general anesthesia. A small incision is made in the umbilicus (belly button) and a long scope with an attached camera and light is inserted. The abdomen is distended with carbon dioxide gas, allowing the surgeon to see into the abdominal cavity. Other small incisions may be made in the lower abdomen to insert other ports through which instruments can be placed to aide with visualization and to perform other maneuvers.

Once visualization of the uterus, ovaries, fallopian tubes, and pelvic peritoneum is achieved, implants of endometriosis can be identified. Common locations include behind the uterus, on the pelvic sidewall, and along the tubes and ovaries. These sites then can be incised or burned. Endometriosis can also cause scarring or adhesions, causing the pelvic structures to be matted together. These adhesions can be taken down via laparoscopy. This is called "lysis" of adhesions.

Large ovarian cysts containing thick chocolate-colored fluid can also be found in patients with endometriosis. These are called endometriomas, and can be surgically removed via laparoscopy as well. Ablating endometriotic implants, taking down adhesions, and removing an endometriotic cyst can provide significant relief of the pain caused by endometriosis.

Once surgery is complete and a diagnosis of endometriosis is made, a strategy for long-term treatment should be considered. Use of a GnRH agonist such as Lupron or Zoladex is effective in treating any remaining endometriosis and contributes to keeping the disease in remission. This is usually done for 6 months. Once this course of therapy is complete, continued treatment with hormones, such as birth control pills or progestin-only therapy, is ideal to prevent recurrence. Another option is to use progestins or birth control pills immediately after the surgery.

Endometriosis can recur once treatment is stopped. The recurrence rate has been reported at 45 percent at 5 years after treatment. For some this can be frustrating and debilitating. Definitive treatment involves a complete hysterectomy with the removal of both ovaries. This is the ultimate treatment of endometriosis; however, the consequence is premature menopause, which leads to other medical issues and concerns. Leaving the ovaries is another option with immediate suppressive treatment to minimize the chance of recurrence. This decision should be made in conjunction with your health care provider once all other options have been tried or at least considered.

Interstitial Cystitis

Interstitial cystitis (IC), also referred to as Painful Bladder Syndrome, is a common cause of chronic pelvic pain in women. The prevalence of this condition is unclear, but it is often underdiagnosed and many women can suffer from this condition for years before it is identified.

IC is a chronic inflammatory condition of the bladder that produces pelvic pain, urinary frequency, urinary urgency, other voiding problems, vulvar or vaginal pain. It can also cause pain with intercourse, as well as severe menstrual-related pain. It is easy to see why this condition is often confused with recurrent urinary tract infections and endometriosis. In many cases women may suffer from both conditions, as well as IC.

The exact cause of this condition is unknown. Research indicates that the protective coating of the bladder has been destroyed. As a result, substances in the urine can seep into the deeper layers of the bladder and irritate the nerve endings. This leads to pelvic pain, urinary frequency, and urgency.

The first step in making the diagnosis is to eliminate other potential causes, such as a bladder infection, malignancy, endometriosis, and pelvic infection. Diagnostic tests for IC exist but are not perfect. The Pelvic Pain and Urgency/Frequency questionnaire asks specific questions that are highly predictive of IC. The potassium sensitivity test (PST) is an in-office test that grades the response to instillation of a potassium solution into the bladder. Women with IC have a dramatic response while women with a normal bladder do not experience any change in sensation. Finally, there's cystoscopy with hydrodistension, which used to be considered the gold standard. However, findings of IC are not consistent and similar findings can be seen in women who do not have symptoms of IC. On the other hand, it is valuable in ruling out bladder cancer as the cause of the problem.

Treatment tends to be multimodal. Elmiron is the only oral agent that is FDA-approved for the treatment of this IC. It should be taken for 3 to 6 months in order to be effective. It is thought to work by rebuilding the protective lining of the bladder. Short-term relief of symptoms can be obtained by instilling soothing agents into the bladder. Dimethylsulfoxide and a cocktail of heparin, sodium bicarbonate, and lidocaine are two examples. They are typically given weekly for 6 to 8 weeks. Use of oral bladder analgesics and anticholinergic agents are helpful in controlling urinary frequency and urgency. The pain can be controlled with the selective use of analgesics. Tricyclic antidepressant agents (amitriptyline or impramine), antiseizure medications (gabapentin), and selective serotonin reuptake inhibitors may also be helpful.

Avoidance of certain trigger foods, such as caffeine, high acidic foods, and potassium-rich foods can provide some relief. Stress and seasonal allergies are triggers for some, who find benefit in stress reduction and use of allergy medications. Sacral nerve stimulation (Interstim) has recently been found to be effective in some women who do not respond to the above listed treatments.

IC is a complex problem and should be managed by a health care provider who is experienced in dealing with chronic pelvic pain in women.

Ovarian Cyst

Cysts on the ovary is a common cause of acute pelvic pain. Cysts typically develop in menstruating women but can also occur in postmenopausal women. A cyst is a fluid-filled structure like a balloon that can enlarge as more fluid accumulates. The size can range from a few millimeters up to 10 centimeters—or larger. The term "cyst" is a general description used for a growth on the ovary. The other term used is "mass," but many find the term cyst is less intimidating. Masses or cysts can also develop within the fallopian tubes. "Adnexal masses" refers to growths in the tube or ovary.

Most ovarian cysts resolve on their own, and those that don't are usually benign (not cancerous). Simple ovarian cysts result from normal ovarian function. They can be found in most women and are a common incidental finding on pelvic imaging. The desire to diagnose ovarian cancer in its earliest state results in an increased surveillance of ovarian cysts. It is important to remember that the incidence of ovarian cancer is around 1 to 2 percent. The lifetime risk of surgery for a suspected adnexal malignancy is 5 to 10 percent and of these only 13 to 21 percent are found to be a cancer.[16]

The ovary is the reservoir of the reproductive cells, called oocytes or eggs. When fertilized by a sperm, a released egg develops into an embryo and then a fetus. The oocytes develop from follicles that are stored in the ovary's stroma (connective tissue). At birth a female infant has over 400,000 follicles. After puberty these follicles are capable of proliferating in an attempt to become a mature egg. Each month a few follicles grow and usually one will mature enough to be released as an egg. The rest will regress.

As the follicles develop they can trap fluid, and this can develop into a cyst. Follicular cysts are the most common type of cyst found. They usually are multiple and small. Once an egg is released (ovulation), the cells at this site continue to proliferate and produce hormones. This proliferation will stop if fertilization doesn't occur. If fertilization does occur the growth continues and produces hormones to support the pregnancy until the placenta is capable of taking over this function. The site of ovulation is called the corpus luteum and a corpus luteal cyst can also occur.

The surface of the ovary can develop inclusion cysts. These are typically quite small, usually only a few millimeters in size. These are a common finding in postmenopausal women.

Finally, benign tumors can develop from any cells of the ovary. They typically do not resolve and will continue to grow, eventually requiring surgical removal. A common type is the dermoid cyst (or mature teratoma), which can grow as large as 15 centimeters or more. Endometriosis on the ovary can grow and swell into a chocolate-colored cyst called an endometrioma. Both kinds of cysts can be managed medically, but sometimes will require surgical resection.

An adnexal mass can also be from the fallopian tubes. Tubal cysts, a hydrosalpinx, or a tubo-ovarian abscess are common conditions that present as adnexal masses. An ectopic pregnancy can also present as a mass, in which case an accurate diagnosis should be made as soon as possible to avoid the life-threatening emergency of a tube rupturing.

Ovarian Cyst Management

Ovarian cysts or adnexal masses may be discovered as a result of pelvic pain or as an incidental finding on routine ultrasound. Occasionally they can cause sudden, acute, severe pain, which may be the result of a twisting of the ovary (called torsion) or a ruptured cyst spilling fluid into the peritoneum and causing significant pain. In this situation surgery may be required, but in most cases there is time to do a proper evaluation of the cause.

Any suspected mass should be evaluated with a complete physical examination, pelvic ultrasound, and a pregnancy test in reproductive-aged women. The first step is to make sure there isn't an ectopic pregnancy. Typically, the ultrasound can provide characterization of the cyst, which will help in determining the next management step. The management is also dependent on the age of the patient, as post-menopausal women have a higher risk of ovarian cancer. A single thin-walled cyst with smooth borders is most likely benign, and two-thirds tend to resolve even in post-menopausal women if their size is less than 10 cm.

Cysts that are described as complex with solid components are more concerning. The presence of other factors can also help the radiologist determine the chance of cancer. A CA 125 test, which looks for the presence of cancer antigen 125 in the blood, is useful in determining the likelihood of an epithelial ovarian malignancy. If a patient's CA 125 is elevated, there is a 98 percent positive predictive value in postmenopausal women compared to 49 percent in premenopausal women. It is not considered useful as a screening test because it is elevated only 50 percent of the time in Stage 1 ovarian epithelial cancers. In addition, benign conditions like endometriosis and leiomyoma (fibroids) can also cause an elevated CA 125 level. Other tumor markers can be used if a germ cell tumor is suspected.

If the tests suggest that the adnexal cyst is benign, the doctor should just suggest observation. Ultrasounds can be done every 6 to 12 weeks to confirm resolution or stability of the cyst. If it isn't growing and there aren't any undesirable symptoms, continued observation is acceptable. Surgery would be recommended if the pain is unmanageable or observation is not possible.

The incidental finding of an ovarian cyst is a common occurrence and there isn't any reason to panic. The vast majority will resolve on their own. You should consider surgery if you are having undesirable pain, if the mass is growing, or if there is a suspected neoplasm (growth). The majority of growths are not cancerous.

Adenomyosis

Heavy and painful periods are typically thought to be due to leiomyoma (uterine fibroids) or abnormal bleeding that happens to all perimenopausal women, but there is another potential explanation: adenomyosis. Traditionally, this condition was not commonly seen as a clinical diagnosis, but this has been changing since recent research indicates that it may be the culprit in more situations than previously thought. Adenomyosis is defined as the benign invasion of the endometrium into the myometrium.

First described in 1860, adenomyosis is a condition wherein the lining of the uterus (endometrium) has somehow started to grow into the muscle of the uterus. It is a similar concept as endometriosis, in which endometrial tissue is growing in places outside the uterine lining. Unlike endometriosis, this causes a diffuse enlargement of the uterus and is sometimes confused with leiomyoma. It can exist is conjunction with fibroids but is a different, distinct histopathologic entity.

Symptoms associated with this condition include heavy bleeding with menstruation (menorrhagia), painful periods, pelvic pain, and pain with intercourse. The cause is unclear but some theories are being studied. Adenomyosis has been noted to be present more often in women who have had a uterine procedure such as a cesarean section, D&C, or myomectomy. Surgical trauma is therefore considered to be the inciting factor that triggers this disorder. Another theory considers the trophoblastic invasion of the placenta into the uterine wall that occurs during pregnancy as a possible initiating factor.

In the past, adenomyosis could only be diagnosed at the time of a hysterectomy when the uterine specimen was examined microscopically. Now ultrasound and magnetic resonance imaging (MRI) can provide detail views of the uterus, allowing for the diagnosis. MRI is the preferred imaging technique because it is much more sensitive (88 percent) and specific (93 percent) in its detection.[18]

The condition appears to be more prevalent in women in their 40s and 50s. This certainly could be because women in that age group are more likely to undergo a hysterectomy where 20 to 47 percent of the uterine specimens are noted to have adenomyosis. Younger women are more likely to be treated conservatively, and detailed MRI imaging is rarely done. In either case the symptoms of heavy bleeding, painful periods, and pelvic pain can be managed with hormonal contraceptive medication, analgesic medications, and other hormonal injections—just as in the treatment of endometriosis. If conservative treatment fails, surgical therapy is the next alternative. In women who wish to preserve their fertility, resection of the involved area has been tried but the efficacy is only about 50 percent.

Adenomyosis is a possible explanation for heavy, painful menses and pelvic pain. The treatment of the condition is like the treatment of endometriosis, dysmenorrhea, and unexplained menorrhagia, so even if you have the condition and are experiencing problems, you are most likely receiving the appropriate treatment. It is worth understanding if you are not having any improvement despite treatment or are considering surgery.

THE BOTTOM LINE

- Chronic pelvic pain is a frustrating problem and the cause can sometimes be difficult to identify.

- Endometriosis and chronic interstitial cystitis/painful bladder syndrome are a common cause of chronic pain, while ovarian cysts usually cause acute pain.
- Consultation with an experienced gynecologist is advised if you are suffering from chronic pelvic pain

Chapter 5

Preventing and Achieving Pregnancy

The reproductive years is the time when most women are sexually active and are at risk of getting pregnant. Women should be aware of issues surrounding conception. Some women have elected to have children but need effective contraception to plan and space their pregnancies. Others may have decided to start a family and have difficulties conceiving. For women who have elected not to reproduce, effective contraception is even more important to avoid unwanted pregnancies. This chapter will focus on contraception and infertility.

Contraception

My colleague and patient Tamara is amazing. She has a busy neurosurgery practice and four boys who are bright, articulate, and well-behaved. I don't know how she does it. She came to see me for some advice. At 36, she's thinking that she might be finished with her family but still holds out a sliver of hope for having a daughter. Her busy schedule makes it difficult to take the pill on time. She wants to know the options.

Long-Acting Reversible Contraception

Are you looking for a birth control that is highly effective, low risk, reversible, and requires little effort to use? Consider a long-acting reversible contraception, such as an intrauterine device or a subdermal implant.

Intrauterine Devices (IUD)

The intrauterine device (or coil) has been in use for over a century. It is a foreign object placed in the uterus through the cervix to prevent pregnancy. It is attached to a string that extends through the cervix, allowing easy removal by pulling the string. It provides contraception through a number of different effects: impaired sperm motility, ovulation prevention, destruction of the ovum, and alteration of the endometrium so that implantation is not possible.

The IUD has a reported effectiveness of more than 99 percent, making it equally effective as permanent sterilization. It can be easily inserted and removed in a doctor's office. The risk of complications is low and can be minimized by appropriate selection of candidates. This is a good option for women who are not good candidates for hormonal contraception and those who want a simple method of contraception but are not ready to undergo a permanent procedure.

In the U.S., there are two types: a hormonal and a copper. The Paragard (the copper T380A IUD) is made of copper and is approved for use up to 10 years. The failure rate is 0.8 out of every 100 women over 10 years, which is comparable to female sterilization. The Mirena contains the hormone levonorgestrel, which is a progestin hormone. It releases the hormone directly into the endometrium at a rate of 20 mcg a day. It is approved for 5 years but continues to release 14 mcg per day during years 5 to 7, so it has possible effectiveness of up to 7 years. Its 1-year failure rate is 0.2 out of every 100 women. This IUD has the additional benefit of decreasing blood loss with menses. Some women don't even have a period because of the progestin. Recently, other progestin IUDs with even lower doses of hormone have come on the market, providing a greater variety of choice. Thus, it is a good treatment option for women with heavy irregular periods, painful periods, and those with endometriosis.[19]

As with all procedures, there are potential risks and undesirable side effects. Expulsion is the major concern, which occurs in 2- to 10 percent of users over one year. The likelihood of expulsion occurs when the IUD is placed immediately postpartum or if it is placed in a uterus with a size outside of the recommend parameters of 6 to 10 centimeters. There is also the potential of uterine perforation at the time of insertion, but this is extremely unlikely, occurring in 1 out of 1000 insertions. Heavy bleeding, prolonged bleeding, and pain are the most common reasons for removal, and this occurs in 1-4 women per 100 users.[20]

The intrauterine device should be entertained by all women who are in a monogamous relationship, who desire effective, easy contraception, but are not yet ready for permanent sterilization. If you elect to use the progestin device there is the bonus of a reduction or even absence of menstrual blood flow.

The Contraceptive Implant

Long-acting reversible contraception includes intrauterine contraceptive devices and contraceptive implants. From a population healthcare perspective, their advantage is the reduction in the unintended pregnancy rates, primarily due to improved compliance. Individuals may appreciate many other advantages, and these methods should be made available to all women. The original subdermal implant, Norplant, is no longer available; however, it paved the way for a much better product: the etonogestrel implant.

Approved by the FDA in 2006, it is currently the only available device of this type in the U.S.

It is a single, rod-shaped subdermal implant that measures 4 centimeters in length and 2 millimeters in diameter. The rod consists of an ethylene vinyl acetate copolymer core filled with 68 mg of etonogestrel surrounded by skin of the same material, which allows for a slow release of the hormone over 3 years. The device is latex-free but not radiopaque or biodegradable. It must be removed once the medication is utilized. The etonogestrel is the active metabolite of desogestrel, which is used in many combination oral contraceptive pills.

Contraception is achieved through the suppression of ovulation. If the egg isn't released, it isn't available for fertilization. The pregnancy rate with this device is 0.05 percent, making it the most effective method of reversible contraception.[19] Other hormonal effects include thickening of the cervical mucus and thinning of the endometrial lining, two situations that also prohibit pregnancy. The effects on menstruation vary but can include a complete cessation of bleeding (amenorrhea), infrequent bleeding, and more frequent or prolonged bleeding. If the latter occurs, the bleeding is usually light but can be annoying. Given the effects on menstruation, the implant could also be used to manage painful periods, endometriosis, adenomyosis, and other menstrual disorders.

The complication rates of insertion and removal are low, but include pain, bruising, bleeding, difficult insertion, unrecognized non-insertion, device breakage, and inability to locate the device at the time of removal. Once it is in place, dissatisfaction with the device tends to be related to side effects. Abnormal bleeding, as mentioned earlier, is the most common undesirable event. Weight gain, acne, headaches, and breast pain are the other complaints. Weight gain occurs in about 6 to 12 percent of users, while the acne appears in

10 to 14 percent.[20] Others may experience improvement in acne or no change at all. Fertility rapidly returns once the device is removed.

The contraceptive subdermal implant should be considered in women who need long-term contraception. It is effective for 3 years, the side effects are minimal, and complication rates are low. An unintended pregnancy is more costly and risky. If you are interested in the implant, take the time to find a health care provider who is trained in the insertion techniques. This will minimize the chance of an adverse event.

Permanent Sterilization

Permanent sterilization should be considered as a birth control option for those who have completed their childbearing or those who have no desire for fertility. The word "permanent" must be emphasized. Even though there are cases where permanent sterilization has been reversed, it is important to have the expectation that this is not reversible. There are methods available that are equally effective but not permanent if there is any doubt.

Permanent sterilization entails the cutting or blocking of the fallopian tubes to prevent the egg and sperm from meeting. This avoids fertilization. (There is an option for permanent sterility in men also, called a vasectomy.) In women, there are many different techniques that have evolved and become more refined over time. Currently tubal occlusion can be performed laparoscopically, immediately postpartum, or with a hysteroscopic approach.

Immediately following delivery, a small incision can be made beneath the umbilicus. The uterus is still enlarged, so the fallopian tubes can be grasped through this small incision. A portion of the tube is removed and then tied to control bleeding. Laparoscopy is a technique using a camera and a small incision in the umbilicus and another in the lower abdomen. Clips or bands can be placed on the tube to obstruct it. The tubes can also be burned during laparoscopy, utilizing a method called electrocoagulation.

The newest method is performed via a trans-cervical route. The Essure procedure, approved for use in 2002, entails placement of a coiled microinsert in the proximal portion of each tube by going through the uterine cavity using a hysteroscope. The implant is 4 cm with a stainless steel inner coil and a nickel titanium outer coil. Over time, the area develops scars, leading to complete obstruction of the tube.

At 3 months, 96 percent of women will have complete obstruction and 100 percent by 6 months. This procedure is done without an incision and can be performed in a doctor's office. It is just as effective as the traditional sterilization techniques as long as appropriate follow-up is completed. The major disadvantage is the need for radiologic confirmation of obstruction 3 to 6 months after the procedure. Interval contraception is required. This procedure is indeed permanent as tubal reversal is impossible.

Permanent sterilization is attractive because it is simple, effective, and minimally invasive. The success rate is generally greater than 99 percent, but varies depending on several factors. A failure of 5.5 per 1000 procedures in the first year is one reported rate. If the procedure fails, then the risk of a tubal or ectopic pregnancy is approximately 32 percent. Overall, the risk of an ectopic pregnancy is much lower in a sterilized woman than a non-sterilized one. Failure of tubal sterilization may be attributed to different causes. Tubal reanastomosis (reconnection) or recanalization (restored flow) can also occur. Failure of equipment and surgical error are also possibilities.

Not all procedures are created equal. The pregnancy rate for postpartum partial salpingectomy is 6.3 pregnancies per 1000 procedures at 5 years. The hysteroscopic implant is the lowest with 1.64/1000, while the bipolar coagulation pregnancy rate is 16.5/1000. The silicone band has a rate of 10/1000, while the spring clips rate is 31/1000. The greatest risk after this procedure is that of ectopic pregnancy. In general, the rate is 7.3 ectopics per 1000 procedures, however this risk is highest in those who had bipolar coagulation with rate of 17 ectopics per 1000 procedures.[22]

Tubal occlusion is an excellent choice for women who have completed their childbearing, especially those who may not be good candidates for other birth control methods. One other important, rarely discussed benefit of tubal occlusion is the decreased risk of ovarian cancer.

It is important to discuss the risks and benefits of permanent sterilization with your doctor. Because not all methods are equal, it is also wise to discuss the appropriate method for you. Serious thought should be given to having it done immediately postpartum if you are certain that you have completed childbearing. Discussion of other available contraception should be a part of this counseling visit. Being informed will allow you to make the choice that is most appropriate for you.

THE BOTTOM LINE

- Long-acting reversible contraceptives, such as an intrauterine device or implant, are highly effective and a good option for women who want a method they don't have to think about.
- Permanent sterilization methods are not the same. Some have a higher failure rate than others.
- Learn about all the available options before making a final decision.

Infertility

Chante's lifelong dream has been to have a family. She had always imagined meeting the man of her dreams, walking down the aisle, carrying a baby, and raising her kids along with a committed partner. But she promised herself that every step had to be ideal, so when her first marriage ended in divorce she was devastated. She remarried 2 years ago, and has been quite happy, so when I see her name on the schedule I assume it's for a new pregnancy visit. I burst into the room but my big smile dissolves as I see the look of disappointment on her face. A single tear slides down her cheek. "It's not happening," she declares and then starts to sob loudly.

The inability to conceive when desired is one of the most difficult challenges for a couple. It creates stress, distress, and can lead to marital strife. The issue is complex and typically there are multiple factors that contribute to infertility. In most cases, resolution of the problem is straightforward. It is important to seek consultation with an appropriate health care provider for assistance, but learning more about the issue can alleviate anxiety and better prepare you for the visit.

Understanding Infertility

Infertility is defined as the failure to conceive after 12 months of regular intercourse in the absence of contraception in a woman less than 35 years of age. The time interval is 6 months in women older than 35. A history of prior pregnancies does not alter the diagnosis. The infertility can be primary or secondary. The term "subfertility" is sometimes used to describe the situation when an actual cause has yet to be identified.

The term "fecundability" describes the probability of conception within 1 menstrual cycle. This rate is about 25 percent in the first 3 months of attempted conception and declines after this. 85 percent of couples will conceive within the first year and 95 percent by 2 years.

The infertility rate in the U.S. is approximately 12 to 18 percent, and 10 percent of women have received some type of fertility services.[23]

There are many potential contributors to infertility. Evaluations have proven that the issue is due to the couple 35 percent of the time, 8 percent it is a male-only factor, and 37 percent female-only. In 5 percent of cases the cause is never identified.[24]

Successful reproduction requires accurate function at every step of the process. It is truly a production line, where malfunction at any stage can affect the end product. The male must have sperm that are adequate in function and number. Coitus must occur at the right time in the menstrual cycle, since the egg is only around for about 2 days per cycle. The cervix and uterus must allow passage of the sperm and the tube must allow passage of the sperm and egg. Once they meet in the tube, fertilization must occur and adequate cell division must commence. The bundle of cells then must travel to the uterus and imbed successfully in the uterine lining.

Male factor infertility can include many issues: no sperm, low sperm, abnormal sperm, or sperm going in the wrong direction. For women, ovulatory dysfunction is usually the problem. Women can have no ovulation, infrequent ovulation, or irregular ovulation. There are many factors that contribute to ovulatory problems. Structural abnormalities, such as tubal obstruction, uterine polyps, fibroids, or adhesions can also prevent the egg and sperm from meeting.

As you can see, the reproductive process is quite complex; the fact that conception occurs in the majority of women is indeed a miracle. If you have a problem, seek the care of an experienced fertility specialist. Be prepared to undergo a comprehensive evaluation and be patient since the suggested test and treatment will be tailored to meet your needs.

Infertility Evaluation

Infertility rates are higher in older couples because female fertility starts to decline each year after 30 and then plummets after 40.

The probability of successful conception is 95 percent at 2 years; however, that doesn't mean that you should wait 2 years before seeking care if you sense there is a problem. You should seek advice if you are under 35 years of age and have had regular intercourse without success for 1 year. If you are over 35 you should seek care after 6 months, and sooner if you are 40. Finally, you should seek care if there are any signs or symptoms that indicate a problem.

A comprehensive history of both you and your spouse should be taken. The history will include medical, surgical, family, and gynecologic history. In-depth questions about your menstrual cycles, history of pain or infections, and coital activity will be asked. Depending on the results, the fertility doctor may suggest that your partner have a detailed physical examination by a urologist. The gynecologist will then perform a detailed physical examination, including a pelvic examination, to see if there are any abnormalities that could indicate a cause for the infertility. For instance, an enlarged thyroid might suggest an endocrine problem or a body mass index >30 might indicate insulin resistance. There are many other potential findings.

There are standard evaluations that may be ordered depending on the findings of the history and physical examination. A semen analysis can provide valuable information about the sperm's anatomy and function. Laboratory tests for the woman may include a thyroid or prolactin check to see if there are endocrine problems that would affect ovulation. A progesterone level taken during the luteal phase of the cycle can confirm if ovulation is occurring. Day 3 follicle stimulating hormone, estradiol, and an antimullerian hormone can indicate if there is a low ovarian reserve within the ovaries. Finally, imaging, such as an ultrasound or hysterosalpingogram can indicate if there is tubal obstruction or other uterine abnormalities. Finally, a laparoscopy might be recommended to further evaluate the female reproductive tract.

Subfertility or infertility is a common problem in couples. A thorough evaluation is required if you want to identify and correct the problem. The tools are available; you must decide how much you are willing to undergo. In a small percentage of cases, a cause is not found and in a fortunate few conceptions occur spontaneously even after they have either undergone therapy, which has failed or have stopped actively trying.

Infertility Treatment

Below is a summary of some of the standard recommendations and treatment of infertility.

Weight Management

Monthly ovulation occurs within a certain range of body weights, and this range can be variable and specific to the individual. There are certain weight extremes, however, that are recognized as unhealthy. A body mass index of less than 19 or greater than 30 are outside of the healthy range. If the body mass index is greater than 40, the concern for health problems is more grave. In many cases these extreme weights can cause amenorrhea or irregular cycles. In either situation, ovulation is not occurring and therefore pregnancy will not be achieved. If you are over- or underweight, then some lifestyle changes would be recommended to get to a healthier body weight, which usually leads to return of ovulation. The additional benefit is that a healthier body means a healthier pregnancy.

Timed Intercourse

Most couples don't realize that the egg is only around for 48 hours and the sperm life is approximately 3 to 5 days. Ovulation occurs exactly 14 days prior to the first day of menstruation. If your cycle is exactly 28 days, ovulation occurs on Day 14, with Day 1 being the first day of bleeding. If you have a 30-day cycle, ovulation occurs on Day 16. If you are trying to conceive, it is best to have intercourse 2 days before ovulation, the day of ovulation and 2 days afterwards. If your cycle interval varies you can extend the time of intercourse to cover those days of probable ovulation. Skipping a day allows time for the potential father to build an adequate volume of semen. Timed intercourse can increase the likelihood of the egg and sperm meeting.

Intrauterine Insemination

This is a process by which the semen is placed directly into the uterus, bypassing the cervix. This procedure is helpful if there is a cervical factor contributing to the infertility. In addition, this process decreases the distance that the sperm must travel and therefore may be helpful in cases where there is decreased sperm motility. It is a straightforward procedure that is relatively inexpensive.

Medications

There are several medications that are used to increase the likelihood of successful pregnancy. Most of the medications are designed to encourage or induce ovulation. Metformin is used in women who have insulin resistance. It was initially designed to treat Type 2 diabetes mellitus. It has also been found to facilitate weight loss in women who are overweight. In either case, it has proven benefits.

There are agents designed to induce ovulation. Selective estrogen receptor modulators are one class. Clomiphene is the most commonly used. It is prescribed for 5 days, usually Days 5 to 9 of the cycle, and is typically successful in inducing ovulation within 3 months if the dose is adjusted accordingly. Aromatase inhibitors are another category that is being utilized. The brain produces gonadotropins, which are the main messengers to the ovary, telling it to produce an egg. These can be given in the form of injections, simulating or supplementing those that should have been produced naturally.

Assisted Reproductive Technologies

Assisted reproductive technologies are utilized when the above have failed or if there are other factors that suggest that this method would be the most efficient. *In vitro* fertilization is a method by which eggs are retrieved and then placed in a dish with the sperm. Because the egg and sperm are placed close to each other, fertilization is highly likely. The dividing cells are then placed in the uterus where implantation can take place. Intra-cytoplasmic sperm injection is a procedure by which sperm are injected into an egg, which is an active method of fertilization.

These methods all have their pros and cons. It is important to have a thorough understanding of the risks, benefits, costs and chances of success prior to making any decisions. Therefore, choosing the right physician is vital. You deserve to have care delivered by an experienced provider so you can achieve your goal in the most efficient and effective way possible.

THE BOTTOM LINE

- Fertilization occurs when a sperm fuses with the egg, and the opportunity for this to occur is only a short period each month.

- It can take up to 2 years to get pregnant in a couple without problems.
- There are numerous reasons for infertility and medical options are available to help you achieve your goal of having a family.

Chapter 6

Perimenopause: The Transition

The period from the mid-thirties to menopause is a time when the quality of the eggs produced by the ovary is decreasing. This is a transitional stage where women are gradually losing their reproductive ability. One hallmark of this time is an irregular menstrual cycle because ovulation is not occurring regularly. This and other problems can contribute to abnormal uterine bleeding. These issues can be managed, especially if anticipated.

Menstrual & Perimenopausal Issues

Nia is highly frustrated. She had finally come off birth control pills at age 37. She and her husband were happy with their 3 girls and he had willingly undergone a vasectomy. But now she is experiencing heavy irregular periods—sometimes twice a month—and other times she skips a couple of months. She is moody and snaps at her husband with the least provocation. She is experiencing significant fatigue and feels bloated. "Doc, you've got to help me. I can't go on like this. I felt better when I was taking birth control pills. How can this be?"

Abnormal Uterine Bleeding

Abnormal uterine bleeding is the most common reason for gynecologic surgery in premenopausal women. Dysfunctional uterine bleeding is another term used to describe this problem. Uterine bleeding is considered to be abnormal if the menses (period) occurs more frequently, lasts longer than usual, or if the amount of bleeding is much heavier than normal.

Periods typically occur every 24 to 35 days and last 5 to 7 days. Average blood loss during this time is usually 80 ml (about 2.7 ounces). More frequent bleeding, longer periods, and blood loss in excess of 100 ml per cycle can lead to anemia, the symptoms of which include lack of energy, fatigue, pica (eating unusual things, mostly non-food item), headaches, palpitations, and fainting. In severe cases, a stroke or heart attack might occur. For many women, this heavy bleeding is accompanied by other bothersome symptoms, such as "labor-like" cramps, back pain, fatigue, bloating, irritability, and difficulty concentrating.

Excessive bleeding can be annoying, distressful, and expensive. Wearing a tampon or pad for long periods and changing them constantly can be uncomfortable, disruptive to one's work and social life, and take a big bite out of one's wallet. Heavy bleeding can also create anxiety over the cause of the abnormal flow.

An evaluation by a health care provider is recommended to determine the cause of the abnormal bleeding and to recommend ways to manage it. The first test should be a pregnancy test; an abnormal pregnancy is a common cause of irregular bleeding. Once this is eliminated as a possible explanation, the next consideration is a malignancy. This is a diagnosis that gynecologists do not want to miss! In women over 35, an endometrial biopsy or dilatation and curettage (D&C) might be recommended to evaluate this possibility. It isn't a frequent occurrence, but an early diagnosis can be lifesaving.

The major cause of abnormal bleeding is usually hormonal or anatomic. A woman might have excessive amounts of estrogen in her blood stream suppressing ovulation and stimulating the lining of the uterus to continue to grow. Once the lining decides to shed, the bleeding is uncontrolled. The excessive estrogen can be produced in the body when there is too much fat tissue, or it can be introduced in the body from hormonal medication such as birth control pills or as environmental contaminants found in foods like hormonally fed beef and chicken.

Anatomical factors include uterine fibroids and endometrial polyps. Fibroids are noncancerous tumors that grow in the muscular uterus. A polyp is a finger-like soft tissue structure that grows in the lining of the uterus. They both interfere with the muscular contraction of the uterus, preventing it from clamping down on the blood vessels and thereby controlling blood loss. They both can also interfere with the phasic growth of the endometrial lining, resulting in dysynchronous (not all at once) shedding.

A comprehensive medical evaluation is needed to discover the cause of the irregular bleeding and to provide effective treatment options. A gynecologist approached by a patient with this problem should take a thorough history and perform a detailed examination. Laboratory and radiological tests might be ordered to assist in the evaluation. Treatment options may include medication or surgery.

Evaluation of Abnormal Uterine Bleeding

The first step in evaluating abnormal uterine bleeding is obtaining a history of the problem. Your health care provider will ask questions related to the timing and duration of the bleeding, and should also inquire about the onset and frequency of menses. Even providing information on the number of sanitary pads or tampons you use is a helpful piece of information. Your doctor will ask about other symptoms, such as fatigue, dizziness, and pain. All of this information will help determine if this problem is posing an immediate threat to your health or if it is disrupting your social or economic well-being.

The next step in the process will include simple in-office tests and a physical examination. Checking a patient's blood pressure and pulse may provide clues to other health problems that might be worsened by the bleeding. For example, a fast heart rate may be an indication of severe anemia. A physical examination can provide clues to other possible medical problems that again may be exacerbated by the bleeding.

A pelvic examination is a targeted evaluation of the uterus. A gynecologist can assess the size of the uterus and the presence of fibroid tumors or other pelvic abnormalities. Other tests taken may include a blood draw to assess the degree of anemia with a hemoglobin or hematocrit (a count of red blood cells). Finally, the gynecologist may request permission to perform an endometrial biopsy, which is a simple procedure designed to obtain a sample of tissue from the lining of the uterus. This tissue is sent to a pathologist—a doctor who studies causes of diseases—who can exam it under a microscope to look for evidence of endometrial cancer or other precancerous changes.

Your physician may recommend further evaluation with imaging tests or outpatient procedures designed to evaluate the uterus further. These tests may include:

- A pelvic ultrasound that can measure the size of the uterus and ovaries. Abnormalities such as fibroid tumors, ovarian cysts, and an abnormally thickened uterine lining can be determined.
- A hysterosonogram is a more specialized evaluation of the lining of the uterus. It is essentially the same as a pelvic ultrasound except a saline solution is injected into the lining of

the uterus to produce a better picture. An endometrial polyp or submucosal fibroid can be diagnosed with this procedure.

- An **MRI** (magnetic resonance imaging) is another way to image the uterus. It can give a more detailed assessment of pelvic structures, including showing fibroids in greater detail. The location and size of these fibroids are more specifically determined. In some cases, this test will be used when the ultrasound images are unhelpful.
- A hysteroscopy is an operative procedure that can be performed in the office or in the operating room. This procedure is performed by dilating the cervix and passing a rigid scope with an attached camera into the uterine cavity. The cavity is distended with a solution to aide with visualization. This procedure allows the gynecologist to inspect the lining of the uterus.
- A scraping procedure called curettage can be performed at the same time to obtain a sample of the endometrium for pathologic evaluation.

The results of these tests can provide the information needed for your doctor to make appropriate treatment recommendations.

Treatment of Abnormal Uterine Bleeding

Abnormal uterine bleeding is the primary reason for surgery and emergency gynecologic visits in the premenopausal woman. In many cases reassurance that there is nothing wrong is all that is required. Assuming there is no evidence of malignancy, the options for treating abnormal uterine bleeding are listed below.

Medications

- Anti-inflammatory and anti-fibrinolytic agents can reduce the amount of blood loss during menses by approximately

30 to 50%. Medications studied include mefenamic acid 500 mg every 8 hours; ibuprofen, 600 mg every 6 to 8 hours; and naproxen, 500 mg twice daily. The anti-fibrinolytic is Tranexamic acid, 1300 mg every 8 hours. These medications should be limited to 5 days.

- Birth controls pills are commonly used to treat abnormal uterine bleeding. They contain a combination of estrogen and progestin hormones. They typically regulate the cycle and result in a shorter and lighter menstrual flow.
- Progestin-only pills can be used alone either in a continuous fashion or for 10 to 14 days of the month. The result is irregular light bleeding or no periods at all.
- Depoprovera is a progestin medication that is delivered as an intramuscular injection. It is given every 12 weeks and, in most cases, the person does not experience any bleeding.
- An intrauterine device delivers progestin directly into the endometrium. The result is a lighter period or, in many cases, completes cessation of menses.

Minor Surgery

- Dilation and curettage (D&C) can provide some relief by simply denuding the lining of the uterus. Used in conjunction with a hysteroscopy, it can also identify abnormal uterine structures such as polyps or fibroids. Polyps can easily be removed at the time of a D&C.
- Hysteroscopic resection of fibroids can be done if there is a fibroid in the lining. This procedure essentially trims away the portion of the fibroid that is growing into the lining of the uterus.
- Ablation procedures are very effective, simple to perform, and pose minimal surgical risk to the patient. They destroy

the lining of the uterus either by heating or freezing. The result is either a normal or lighter period or no period.

- Uterine fibroid embolization is a procedure performed by an interventional radiologist. Small amounts of inert material are injected into the uterine artery to obstruct the blood supply to the uterus, resulting in fibroid shrinkage over time.

<u>Major surgery</u>

- Myomectomy is a surgical procedure designed to remove fibroids from the uterus. It is done either via a laparotomy, which involves a large incision on the abdomen, or laparoscopically, meaning it is done using small incisions during which a lighted camera and long slender instruments are placed to perform the procedure. Once the fibroids are removed, sewing the edges of the uterus together repairs the defect.

- Hysterectomy is a procedure in which the uterus is removed. This is the ultimate cure for abnormal bleeding. The ovaries can be left in place. This can be done through an abdominal incision, vaginally, or laparoscopically.

- Women who smoke and are over the age of 35 should not use hormonal therapies. Women with a history of a heart attack, stroke, and deep venous blood clots should also avoid these medications. Caution should also be taken in women with multiple medical problems, especially those with a history of diabetes and hypertension.

- There are also certain reasons why an ablation procedure shouldn't be performed. Your doctor can determine if you are a candidate for this procedure. When considering surgery, an individual's health status should be carefully examined for potential issues. Some women will be at an increased risk of problems such as heart attack, stroke, infection, and deep venous thrombosis.

THE BOTTOM LINE

- Abnormal uterine bleeding is a common problem in women, especially after their mid-thirties.
- There are many options for managing heavy periods and these should be considered to avoid developing severe anemia.
- You should seek care if you are experiencing excessive bleeding with your periods.

Breast Disorders

I enter the exam room to find a very anxious Farrah clutching her gown close to her chest. "Hi Farrah," I say cheerfully and take a seat on the stool in front of her. "I think I have breast cancer," she says fearfully. I reach out and grasp her hand. "Tell me why you say this?" It turns out she had gone to a breast cancer awareness talk and had started doing her breast self-examination and found a lump. Farrah was only 26 years old and her risk of cancer was very low. On examination, I found a smooth, fluctuant lump. I sent her for a breast ultrasound that very same day and it turned out to be a simple cyst.

Evaluating Your Breast

Breast pain, lumps, or changes in a breast's appearance can be indications of a problem. Experiencing any of these tends to cause a great deal of distress, and many women are uncertain what should be done. Some problems should prompt you to see your doctor immediately while others can be monitored for a short time to see if they resolve.

Breast problems generally present in a handful of ways. Breast pain is the most common symptom and can either be cyclic, occurring just before the period, or constant. Cyclic pain typically occurs 1 week before the period and usually resolves with the onset of the period. This happens due to stimulation of the breast tissue by the increased estrogen levels that occur just before menstruation. The drop-in estrogen levels that trigger the period leads to resolution of the breast pain. Even though this is uncomfortable, it is normal. Constant breast pain, however, is more concerning and may be an indication of a greater problem.

A breast mass or lump can be found during a self–breast exam or by a doctor when she does a clinical exam. The lump's presence may be painful or without pain. Sometimes lumps may be associated with pain and occur 1 to 2 weeks before the period and then resolve. This is most likely a breast cyst, a result of the estrogen stimulation. If it resolves, there isn't any concern for a more serious problem; however, it is important to continue regular self-examination. There are multiple causes of lumps, so further imaging tests are usually recommended when the lump persists.

Another symptom is nipple discharge. The discharge can be clear, milky, green, or dark-colored. The discharge can come from one or both breasts. If the discharge is from one side only then it may indicate a local problem with that breast. If the discharge is milky in appearance and/or comes from both breasts it is usually a reflection of a hormonal problem, such as an elevated prolactin. This is most likely the case in women who are pregnant, recently delivered, or recently stopped nursing.

No matter the problem, the goal from a physician's perspective is to relieve the symptoms, make sure it isn't cancer, and determine what this says about your future cancer risks. Certain breast lesions indicate a greater risk of breast cancer. In addition, there are other factors that can place someone at higher or lower risks.

Women who are at higher-than-average risk of breast cancer have one or more of the following factors:

- A family history of breast cancer, especially in first-degree relatives, such as a parent or sibling
- Are postmenopausal
- Have undergone hormone replacement therapy, especially if they did so for longer than 5 year
- Have never been pregnant
- Experienced early onset of menstruation
- Had their first pregnancy at a late age
- Experienced late menopause

Women who are at lower risk of breast cancer generally:

- Breast fed for longer than 3 months
- Have had multiple pregnancies and deliveries
- Experienced premature menopause
- Experienced other factors that may have interrupted menstrual cycles

It is important to know your status. Are you at a higher or lower risk of developing breast cancer? The answer to this question should dictate how vigilant you should be with recommended screenings and how urgently you should see a physician if you develop a breast problem.

Benign Breast Disorders

Breast lesions or changes are a cause for great concern. They can be an incidental finding on breast imaging or detected during a self–breast exam. They can even be found by the doctor on routine examination. In either case, the first question that pops into a woman's head is: "Is this breast cancer?" The answer is usually no; however, the woman will generally go through weeks of tests and waiting before arriving at the answer. The section will describe the non-cancerous problems that are not associated with an increased risk of developing breast cancer.

Breast lesions are classified based on their potential for changing and developing into breast cancer. The category that is not associated with an increased risk of breast cancer development is described as non-proliferative breast disorders. Older terms used to describe these problems were fibrocystic changes, fibrocystic disease, or mammary dysplasia. Women with these problems are at no higher or lower risk of developing breast cancer than women without these problems.

The different categories are described below but breast cysts are the most commonly known.

Breast Cysts

Breast cysts are fluid-filled structures that are round or ovoid in shape. They occur in the terminal breast ducts. They can be solitary or multiple and their size may fluctuate. On imaging, the cyst may be described as simple, complicated, or complex. The complex types are associated with an increased risk of cancer.

Cysts can be affected by hormonal fluctuations, so they can appear during breast development, breast involution (shrinkage) in perimenopausal women, and menstrual cycle changes.

Cysts may present with either sudden pain associated with a lump or as an incidental finding on a mammogram. Sometimes the breast lump is small and not painful but may persist or fluctuate in size throughout the cycle.

Proliferative Breast Disorders

This is the second category of breast disorders. They are associated with a slightly higher risk of developing breast cancer. Women with these problems have a 1.5 to 2 times higher risk of developing cancer in their lifetimes compared to women who do not have this problem. The increased risk is slight, so no special preventative measures are recommended.

Histologically, these lesions are described as proliferative tissue without any atypical changes. This means there is a low risk of developing into cancer. The disorders that fall into this category are described below, with the most commonly recognized is fibroadenoma.

Fibroadenoma

A fibroadenoma is a firm, mobile mass that is usually found on clinical examination. It tends to occur in women ages 15 to 35. The tumor responds to estrogen stimulation as evidenced by the fact that it increases in size during pregnancy or in women on estrogen therapy and regresses during menopause. There can be one or multiple lesions, and they may vary in size.

Ultrasound imaging usually reveals a dense solid tumor that is histologically composed of glandular and fibrous tissue. Even though there are characteristic findings on imaging, biopsy to obtain a tissue sample is recommended when one is found for the first time to be certain of the diagnosis. The tissue sample can be obtained with a core biopsy using a local anesthetic or complete excision to remove the entire lesion. There are pros and cons of each method. The histopathology (examination of the tissue under the microscope) will reveal if the cells are complex or simple. This information, along with a family history or the presence of proliferative changes, can indicate whether there is an increased risk of developing cancer in the future. If the tissue is simple, there isn't an increased risk. Once a clear tissue diagnosis is obtained, future occurrences can be managed appropriately.

Ductal Hyperplasia

This is a condition usually found on biopsy. Microscopic findings indicate an increased number of cells within the usual ductal space. The cell features are benign; however, the mere presence of these increased numbers of cells indicates a slightly increased risk of breast cancer compared to normal.

Papillomas

These appear as masses or nodules found on exam or during mammographic imaging. They can sometimes cause nipple discharge. There can be a single papilloma or multiple. The papillary cells of a cyst wall overgrow and fill the lumen (inside space) of the cyst. These growths can contain cells that are atypical in appearance, or even malignant cells that haven't yet grown past the basement membrane layer—this is referred to as being "in-situ." Because of this potential, any imaging that suggests the presence of a papilloma should be followed with surgical excision. The final histopathologic findings will dictate further management.

Sclerosing Changes

Sclerosing adenosis or complex sclerosing lesions may look like a mass or a suspicious finding on mammography. These lesions should be biopsied to have a clear histologic diagnosis. The complex lesions should undergo complete excision because of the potential to develop into cancer over time or an increased risk of cancer being found in the excised specimen.

The lesions in these groups require a biopsy or excision to determine the correct diagnosis. The reassuring point is that once the tissue is removed, you can rest easy that it is out and you have a clear answer on what caused the problems. Certainly, there is risk of surgery, including scarring, making future evaluation difficult and causing damage to the breast duct system. But the risks are worth it to provide peace of mind and to ensure there isn't a malignancy.

<u>Atypical Hyperplasia and Other Breast Lesions</u>

Atypical hyperplasia is a condition in which cells are undergoing changes that are likely to develop into cancer over time. In the breast, these changes can occur in the ducts or the breast lobes. If the changes occur in the epithelial cells of the ducts, it is called "atypical ductal hyperplasia." "Atypical lobular hyperplasia" describes the changes to the epithelial cells of the breast lobes. The lesions have features like carcinoma in-situ and can be multi-focal lesions.

These conditions are of grave concern because of the associated risk of breast cancer. A woman with either of these conditions has 3.7 to 5.3 times increased risk of developing cancer compared to normal. The cumulative lifetime risk of developing breast cancer over 30 years is close to 35 percent. Even more frustrating is the fact that the cancer can develop in a location remote from the hyperplastic lesion, even in the other breast.

Given this known increased risk of cancer, more frequent surveillance is required. In addition, other preventative factors can be considered. Yearly mammograms and twice-yearly breast examinations are suggested. The doctor's recommendations may also include a regular breast ultrasound. Of course, any suspicious finding should be immediately biopsied or excised.

Women with this condition should avoid hormone replacement therapy and birth control pills. Other preventative measures may be recommended; those are dependent on family history, personal history, and the presence of other risk factors for breast cancer.

There are medications available to reduce the chance of developing breast cancer. These include selective estrogen receptor modulators, such as tamoxifen and raloxifene, or aromatase inhibitors. In-depth counseling with an experienced health care provider is highly recommended before electing to use such medications.

Other breast disorders that are not associated with an increased risk of breast cancer include:

- Lipoma: a mass composed of mature fat cells
- Fat necrosis: an area of liquefied fat that can result from trauma, surgery, or other medical problems
- Galactocele: cystic fluid collection that results from an obstructed milk duct
- Hamartoma: a mass containing glandular, adipose, and fibrous tissue
- Adenoma: benign epithleial cell tumor

There are a number of breast problems that can result in a palpable mass or an abnormal finding on imaging studies. The majority are benign and do not indicate an increased risk of developing breast cancer. These signs should, however, initiate further evaluation to confirm the cause since early breast cancer detection is the key to cure.

THE BOTTOM LINE

- Most breast lumps are not cancerous.
- Breast cysts and fibroadenomas are the most common causes of breast lumps.

- Evaluation of breast abnormalities should be done immediately, however, to increase the chance of early detection in the unlikely event that cancer is present.

Other Health Concerns

Obesity

Uma has always been somewhat overweight but after each pregnancy she put on more weight and struggled to return to her pre-pregnancy level. Now, after her fourth child, she came to see me for an examination. Her body mass index is 45. "Uma, I'm worried about you. Your weight is now in a range that puts you at higher risk for developing serious medical problems. Can we talk about it?" She agreed and we had a long conversation about her diet, exercise routine, and medical care. After ordering several tests, I referred her to see a bariatric specialist with test results in hand.

What is obesity?

Society is obsessed with weight loss and fitness, but why? From a superficial perspective, it seems to be about aesthetics, but when you delve deeper you find it's a response to the alarming statistics that have serious implications for the public's health. The prevalence of obesity has risen sharply in the past decades and now has reached epidemic proportions. Obesity has become one of the top social concerns of our day. But what is obesity and why is it a problem? In this section, we will discuss the concerns and what you can do to stay healthy.

Obesity, as defined by Merriam Webster, is "a condition characterized by the excessive accumulation and storage of fat in the body." This clearly describes the condition, but this also covers being overweight as well. The science of medicine has a more specific definition for this condition and it is based on health risks. They use the measure of body mass index (BMI) to classify the conditions of overweight, obesity and morbid obesity.

The body mass index attempts to adjust for differences in height so weight alone is not used as the measure. It is calculated by dividing the weight in kilograms by the height in meters squared. The inability to adjust for muscle mass limits it from being able to accurately classify everyone but it is a convenient way to categorize groups in general. It is an imperfect test since it does not consider the contribution to the overall weight made by muscle and bones. It is a known fact that certain ethnic groups have denser bones. In addition, more muscular women may fall into a higher BMI category that gives the false impression of an unhealthy weight when they in fact may be healthier than the average person. Finally, it is important to point out that some women might fall into the overweight category but may be perfectly healthy. Until there is a better tool available for wide spread use, BMI is the most objective measure.

In adults, a BMI of 18.5 to 25kg/m^2 is healthy. Overweight is defined as a BMI of 25 to 29.9, while obesity is defined as a BMI more than 30. An individual with a BMI greater than 40 has morbid obesity. Those defined as overweight are at low risk for poor health outcome while the obese group is at moderate risk. Those with morbid obesity are at high risk of poor health outcomes.

These categories are designed to assist with counseling and treatment option. Individuals who are at high risk need urgent, aggressive interventions to correct the problem before they encounter life-threatening health issues. Those with simple obesity may require urgent intervention if there are other factors that increase the risk of poor health outcome.

Another less commonly discussed measure is waist circumference. A waist circumference of more than 40 inches (102 cm) in men and more than 35 inches (88 cm) in women is concerning. In this situation, the risks of cardio-metabolic problems are quite high. This includes hypertension, heart disease, diabetes, elevated lipids, and other vascular diseases.

Classifying the degrees of obesity provides the health community with a standard way of communicating, studying the consequences of obesity, and counseling patients on their risks and recommended interventions. Individuals can use this information to adjust their lifestyles to manage their weight before it reaches a point where there are health risks.

How big is the problem?

Obesity has become a worldwide epidemic, affecting 2.1 billion people. It is predicted that 50 percent of the world's population will be overweight or obese by 2030 if the current trend persists. It is more prevalent in developed countries where food is abundant and the lifestyle doesn't require extensive physical activity. The concern about obesity is not the condition itself but the consequences. Epidemic proportions of obesity translate to epidemic proportion of health problems and this is preventable.

Worldwide, 37 percent of men and 38 percent of women are obese. In the United States, approximately 35 percent of adults are obese and one-third of children are overweight or obese. Morbid obesity (BMI >40 kg/m^2) had a reported prevalence of 6 percent in 2009/2010. This information is supported by self-reported and measured data. The prevalence of obesity increased by over 50 percent from 1988 to 1994 to 2007/2008, but has been stable from 2003/2004 until 2011/2012.[12]

Overweight and obese individuals have a higher risk of mortality and morbidity compared to those of normal weight. Individuals with a BMI of 22.5 to 25 kg/m^2 have the lowest mortality rate of all groups. Those with a BMI over 30 have a 2- to 3-fold increase in risk compared to those with a normal BMI. There is a 30 percent increase in risk for additional health issues for every 5 kg/m^2 gained. For individuals over the age of 50 who are obese, there is a higher death rate for all causes. Obese individuals have a 1.4-fold increase in death from heart disease and stroke, while the risk is 2 times greater from diabetes. Eighty percent of all cases of adult onset diabetes (Type 2 diabetes) are due to obesity. Excessive body weight causes over 25 percent of cases of hypertension, and there is a known association of obesity with cancers of the breast, endometrium, colon, and others.

Another scary statistic relates to life expectancy. The life expectancy is 6 to 7 years less in an obese individual compared to those with a normal BMI. Overweight individuals live 3 to 4 years less. This is worsened by the presence of other risk factors. Those who smoke and are obese live 13 to 14 years less than those of normal body mass index.

There are also financial consequences of obesity. According to the CDC, the cost of obesity is $147 billion/year. The annual cost of healthcare expenditures is 25 percent greater in those with a BMI of 30 to 34.9 kg/m^2 and 44 percent greater among those with a BMI higher than 35 kg/m^2 compared to those with BMI of 20 to 24.9 kg/m^2. In addition, those who are overweight or obese are 2 times more likely to draw disability and take twice as much sick leave as those of normal weight. This further supports the fact that obesity contributes to poor health.

The good news is that there is something that can be done. Overweight and obese individuals who are fit have a similar death risk as those fit individuals of normal weight. Exercising and a healthy lifestyle, including diet, makes a significant difference. So, if you haven't started, now is a good time to begin a regular exercise program and begin a nutritious diet. Do it for yourself and your family.

<u>What causes obesity?</u>

There are theories that imply a predisposition to obesity based on "in utero" exposure. Pregnancy conditions can affect a fetus's medical future. Infants born to mothers who are diabetic or who gain excessive weight during pregnancy are at a higher risk of developing obesity as an adult. Other pregnancy factors include high pre-pregnancy weight and smoking. Breastfed infants are at lower risk of becoming obese. A mother's care of herself and her baby during pregnancy and immediately post-delivery play a role in the risk of obesity in the future.

A lot of women note that pregnancy seems to be the tipping point for when weight gain becomes an issue. It is easy to gain excessive weight during pregnancy and more difficult to return to a normal weight postpartum. The challenges are many, but typically are due to lack of time or motivation for physical activity. The weight gain becomes compounded over subsequent pregnancies resulting in obesity over time. Women who breast-feed their babies tend to return to a normal weight quicker and find that weight loss is much easier.

There are other life phases and events that contribute to weight gain. Menopause is a classic time. A woman's metabolism slows down even more and losing weight is a challenge. Weight loss regimens that worked in the past are not as effective and many struggle to even maintain a stable weight. The transitions from childhood to adolescence and to adulthood are other times women note challenges with weight.

There are also medications and certain medical conditions that contribute to weight gain—either directly or indirectly. Medical conditions such as hypothyroidism and Cushing's disease are examples of endocrine disorders that manifest with weight gain and obesity. Drugs used for depression, diabetes, and epilepsy are also notable for contributing to weight challenges.

Life is full of transitions and phases, many times contributing to weight gain and difficulty maintaining a healthy lifestyle. You should recognize these transition points and work even harder during these intervals to manage your weight, recognizing that this effort will be rewarded in the future. Establishing a healthy lifestyle now, which includes regular exercise and a nutritious diet, will help you manage the challenges that may accompany these life events.

Lifestyle Contributes to Obesity

The causes of obesity are many and certain life events increase the risks of weight gain. The events include intrauterine factors, pregnancy, menopause, medical problems, and certain medications. These factors predispose individuals to weight challenges and may even contribute further to an existing weight management issue. However, the simple answer to the question posed is LIFESTYLE. The lifestyle of western society and developed countries is the primary factor that contributes to this worldwide epidemic.

Body weight reflects muscle mass, fat storage, and water. Weight gain is due to either an increase in the storage of fat or an increase in muscle mass. It is the storage of excessive fat that is a concern, and that is the primary reason for individuals being overweight or obese. Food is a source of energy that the body utilizes to perform its functions. The greater the activity, the more energy is required to fuel this activity. A competitive athlete burns more energy per day than a regular working person.

Energy is measured in calories. The body burns what it needs from the daily intake of food. If there are additional calories left over, this is stored by the body, usually as fat. If the body receives fewer calories than it needs to burn energy, then it will utilize the stored energy sources. Simply put, excessive calorie intake equals increased storage and lower calorie intake leads to utilization of stored energy sources and subsequent weight loss.

Most individuals lead a sedentary lifestyle, meaning they are not physically active. Their work doesn't require much activity and yet they continue to supply their bodies with more fuel than they need. This leads to gradual weight gain, such that 19 percent of women and 30 percent of men become overweight within 4 years and 5 to 9 percent become obese. Over a 30-year period, 50 percent of individuals become overweight and 25 to 30 percent become obese. This is because we don't adjust our eating habits to meet the energy needs of our body. Regular exercise is becoming more of a habit and is likely the reason that the prevalence of obesity has stabilized in the U.S. over the past decade. This habit needs to be adopted by many more.

In our society, food is being used for more than just an energy source. It has become a source of entertainment, socialization, and even therapy. We eat for taste, and the enjoyment of food drives much of the excessive calorie intake. Much of our socialization revolves around food: going out to dinner with friends or on a date, holiday meals, and even eating while enjoying other entertainment, such as at the movies or sports events. The availability of cheap, convenient, calorie-rich foods such as those found at fast food restaurants has made this even worse. We have developed bad eating habits and, unfortunately, the more you indulge in these foods, the more your body seems to crave them. The other source of useless calories comes from the consumption of beverages. They are useless because they don't provide any valuable nutrients. Sodas, juices, and alcohol are a few examples.

More than 60 percent of Americans say they are attempting to lose weight, however only 20 percent are consuming fewer calories and/or exercising at least 150 minutes per week. The solution is simple, but the actualization is difficult. The key to weight control is minimizing the storage of energy in your body. This can be managed by either consuming only what you need to fuel your body or burning more calories to match your daily consumption. The adjustments in calories consumed and physical activity depends on whether you are trying to lose weight or maintain your current weight. Weight management is the most important factor in maintaining good health, and you are in complete control of this.

Weight Management

Weight management begins with an assessment of your current state. Are you overweight or obese? You should measure your body mass index (BMI). If your BMI is 25 to 29.9 you are classified as overweight. If your BMI is greater than 30, you are categorized as obese. If it is greater than 40, you are described as morbidly obese.

The next step is to evaluate your calorie intake and expenditure. Do you exercise? How much? The intensity and duration of exercise helps you determine your energy expenditure. Finally, what do you eat and how much? A food diary is a good way to monitor your intake. Once you have done this for a few days, you can calculate the number of calories you take in per day. There are websites, smart phone applications, watches, and devices that can assist with these measurements.

Now you can start setting goals. Your goals should be SMART: specific, measurable, attainable, realistic, and timely. You didn't gain weight overnight, so it won't come off overnight. Depending on your status, you may focus on the diet aspect or the exercise aspect. It would be advisable to do both; however, the most important step is to get started. Set a goal and, once this has been achieved, set another one. One example may be to exercise 4 times per week for the next 4 weeks. This meets the SMART criteria. Upon examining your food diary, you may discover that you drink a great deal of soda. Another goal might be to drink only water for the next 4 weeks.

You should determine how many calories you need per day based on your activity level and aim to consume fewer if weight loss is your goal. There are smart phone apps that will calculate the number of calories needed to achieve your goal once you put in the required information. There are also some simple interventions that can be taken. Eliminate or severely limit all useless calories, such as alcohol, sodas, candy, chips, and other items that are usually consumed for taste. Educate yourself about nutrition and what is required to fuel your body. Focus on providing your body with ideal fuels, such as lean meats, fruits, vegetables, and grains, and avoiding simple carbohydrates, excessive amounts of food, and those with a high fat content.

Regular exercise has benefits beyond weight loss. It can lower your blood pressure, improve your lipid profile, and help control diabetes. It makes your bones and muscles stronger, improving coordination and minimizing bone loss. It can help boost your mental state and in general helps you feel better. Individuals who exercise on a regular basis have a longer life expectancy.

The best approach is to incorporate exercise into your daily routine by taking up a hobby that you enjoy, like tennis, running, martial arts, biking, or regular walks. The more you do, the more you can do, and the more you will want to do. Start slow and gradually increase. Set SMART goals.

Treatment of Obesity

Immediate intervention is required and the solution is simple: weight management. Since this is a public health problem, the burden of intervention falls on all: government, schools, healthcare providers, employers, and individuals. Many national programs have been put in place in the U.S., and ongoing efforts are apparent. This is probably the explanation behind the stabilization of the prevalence of obesity in the U.S. The government and schools can continue to provide education on proper nutrition and physical activity while putting measures in place to encourage compliance with these recommendations. Employers can do the same. Healthcare providers need to focus more attention on prevention, rather than treatment. Individuals can and should take control of their own health and the health of their families.

Health care researchers have provided risk categories for those who are overweight and obese. These categories help determine the degree of intervention required based on the risk of adverse events in the future. Individuals at low risk include normal weight and those who are overweight (BMI of 25 to 29.9) but healthy. Individuals at moderate risk are overweight with other risk factors (such as heart disease, smoking, or hypertension) and those who have a BMI of 30 to 34.9. Individuals are high risk if their BMI is 35 to 40 or 30 to 34.9 with other risk factors. Finally, individuals with a BMI greater than 40 are at very high risk.

Low-risk individuals should receive education and counseling on physical activity and proper nutrition. This provides them with the information they need to maintain a normal weight throughout the course of their lives. Ideally, this education would be a part of a regular school curriculum and provided at all healthcare encounters. Those at moderate risk should have weight loss/management interventions that include education, diet modification, implementation of regular exercise, and behavior modification if required. They can also be considered for medication therapy if the initial interventions are not effective. Individuals at high risk and very high risk should have aggressive interventions, which include the above, but also medications, lifestyle interventions, and bariatric surgery as a final option.

Medical Management

Diet, regular exercise, and behavior modifications are effective in select groups, but for those with obesity other interventions may be required. Medications and surgery are readily available options for managing obesity and morbid obesity, but they are not without risks. Individuals who have a BMI more than 30 or who have a BMI of 27 to 29 but who have certain medical conditions are considered candidates for medical management.

Drugs are not a permanent solution for weight management but an option to initiate weight loss and/or to supplement the efforts of diet and exercise. In addition, the use of many currently available drugs comes with a number of concerns, including limited effectiveness, side effects, the potential for adverse events, and cost. All of these factors should be taken into consideration when electing to utilize medication to assist with weight loss. Individuals are candidates for medication use if they are obese or if they are overweight with medical conditions that place them at high risk of serious outcomes in the future and other interventions have not been effective.

Drugs shouldn't be used in isolation, but as an adjunct to regular exercise, proper diet, and behavior modification. An effective weight loss program should show a drop-in body weight by 5 to 10 percent because this is the point where health benefits are seen. Expected weight loss usually exceeds 2kg per month (1 lb per week) dropping to more than 5 percent below baseline weight at the 3- to 6-month period. Drug trials using both drug and behavior modification view a weight loss of 10 to 15 percent as a good response and more than 15 percent as an excellent response.

There are 2 drugs available that have a proven efficacy and a reasonable safe profile: orlistat and lorcaserin. Orlistat is the recommended first line medication. It inhibits the enzyme pancreatic lipase, thus preventing the digestion of fat. The dose is 120 mg three times a day. Drug trials showed an average weight loss of 5 to 10 kg in those taking this drug compared to 3 to 6 kg for control subjects. Typical side effects are related to the gastrointestinal tract and include nausea, gassiness, flatus, and loose and oily stools. It can be used up to 2 to 4 years and generally has no other major effects. The only concern of note is that it may decrease the absorption of fat-soluble vitamins, so supplements are encouraged.

Lorcaserin is a serotonin agonist with efficacy equivalent to Orlistat that works by decreasing the appetite. It should be considered for individuals who have intolerable side effects on Orlistat. The dose is 10 mg twice daily, and reported side effects include headache, nausea, and back pain. Long-term safety data is limited.

Other drugs have been used. It is best to consult with a bariatric specialist before starting any drug regimens for weight loss.

Surgical Management

The appropriate term for obesity surgery is bariatric surgery. It is the most effective form of weight loss available and is recommended for individuals with morbid obesity and/or individuals with a BMI greater than 35 who suffer from other chronic medical conditions, such as diabetes. Outcomes show a 20 to 30 percent weight loss after 1 to 2 years, and partial or full resolution of Type 2 diabetes, hypertension, hypercholesterolemia and obstructive sleep apnea.

Bariatric procedures work by either restricting the amount of food that can be consumed or by contributing to malabsorption of the food that is consumed. Some procedures have both effects. The first procedure was performed in the 1950s and was a malabsorptive-type procedure designed to inhibit absorption of nutrients. It led to significant nutritional problems, including vitamin deficiencies, diarrhea, and protein–calorie malnutrition. This specific type of procedure is no longer performed but it served as the springboard for more effective procedures.

Current technology and surgical advancements have given birth to a number of simple, effective, minimally invasive bariatric procedures. Most surgeries can be performed either via the traditional open route or by laparoscopy. In 2003, 20 percent of cases were laparoscopic. This increased to 90 percent by 2008, which has resulted in fewer complications and faster recovery times. It is now one of the fastest growing surgical subspecialties, with over 340,000 procedures performed annually worldwide, approximately 200,000 of those performed yearly in the U.S.

Individuals who meet the criteria for weight loss surgery should seek treatment through a recognized bariatric program. The key to a successful and satisfactory outcome is extensive education and counseling provided by a bariatric team. This should cover all aspects of the surgery: expectations of outcomes, nutrition, and lifestyle changes required to facilitate long-term success, including psychological assessment and counseling. The other major component of the team is a skilled and experienced surgeon. The American Society for Metabolic and Bariatric Surgery is one source for finding qualified providers.

If you suffer from chronic diseases related to obesity, there are options for getting back on a healthful path. Talk with your doctor to see if bariatric surgery is an option for you. If your doctor is not knowledgeable, search for a bariatric and weight management program in your area. You can have a consultation visit where information is provided. Many individuals who have gone through this procedure say it was a life-changing experience. It may also be a life-saving one.

Types of Bariatric Surgery

Bariatric procedures are categorized as restrictive procedures, malabsorptive procedures, or a combination of both. The restrictive procedures decrease the capacity of the stomach, thus limiting the amount of food a person can consume and thus their caloric intake. The advantage of these procedures is that weight loss is gradual. Malabsorptive procedures work by decreasing the effectiveness of nutrient absorption by shortening the length of the functional small intestine. This is done either by a physical bypass of the small intestine or by diverting the biliopancreatic secretions, which are used to facilitate absorption. This results in significant and more rapid weight loss but has a higher probability of causing nutritional deficiencies.

Roux-en-Y gastric bypass (**RYGB**) is the most commonly performed procedure. It represented 65 percent of all bariatric procedures in 2003 but had decreased to 47 percent by 2011. It is both a restrictive and malabsorptive procedure. The procedure creates a small gastric pouch and bypasses a portion of the small intestine, limiting the amount of calories absorbed. The expected weight loss after 2 years is approximately 70 percent.

Laparoscopic adjustable gastric banding (**LAGB**) involves the placement of a tight adjustable prosthetic band on the entrance to the stomach. It is a restrictive procedure and is the least invasive procedure in this group. It accounted for 24 percent of the procedures in 2003, though its use dropped to 18 percent in 2011. It has the lowest mortality rate of all the bariatric procedures and there is usually a

50 to 60 percent weight loss at 2 years. However, it requires more revisions and has a higher rate of individuals regaining the lost weight.

Sleeve gastrectomy (SG) involves the partial removal of the stomach, restricting the volume of food that can be consumed. In 2011, it was the second most commonly performed bariatric procedure, representing 28 percent of all procedures performed. It is much safer and easier than a RYGB and has a weight loss of about 60 percent at 2 years. If the desired weight loss is not achieved with this procedure it can be easily converted into a gastric bypass or other procedure.

Other procedures include the biliopancreatic diversion with duodenal switch (BPD/DS) and the mini gastric bypass. They are both a combination of restrictive and malabsorptive procedures. The BPD/DS is a complex procedure with 70 to 80 percent weight loss at 2 years and is performed in only a few centers in the U.S. The mini gastric bypass is a modification of the loop gastric bypass, but much easier than the RYGB. It is also safe and easily revised, reversed, and converted. Long-term data is limited but it appears to have a success rate of 50 percent weight loss at 18 months.

Outcomes of Bariatric Surgery

Bariatric surgery is the most effective method of weight loss and is an excellent option for individuals with morbid obesity or who are obese and suffer from medical conditions attributable to obesity. Of course, every intervention has possible after effects and complications.

Individuals can also expect partial or complete resolution of their obesity-related medical conditions, such as hypertension, diabetes, elevated cholesterol, and obstructive sleep apnea.

Early complications from these procedures include bowel obstruction, leaks from the intestinal anastomosis (connection) sites, infections, injury to internal organs, thromboembolic events, return to surgery, and breathing difficulties. Heart attacks and strokes can also occur due to the stress of the surgery. There are many factors that affect the risks of these outcomes, including the surgeon's skill, individual factors (obesity increases the risks of all these problems), and adherence to pre- and post-surgical protocols designed to decrease these events.

Long-term problems include intestinal ulcers, gallstones, kidney stones, stenosis at the stomach outlet, depression, and abdominal pain. Dumping Syndrome is also a potential problem. It is a condition where ingested food passes rapidly through the digestive tract before adequate absorption of nutrients can occur. This leads to chronic diarrhea and results in malnutrition. The possibility of regaining all of the weight also exists. Extensive pre-surgical counseling and follow-up after surgery is designed to prepare individuals for these outcomes and provide interventions as needed. In addition, behavioral modifications should be discussed before the surgery. Individuals should plan to adhere to recommended diet and exercise to maintain a normal weight.

The risk of adverse events and mortality (death) are much lower now than in the past. The 30-day mortality rate is less than 1 percent, and the majority of deaths are due to pulmonary embolism, cardiac events such as an infarction, respiratory failure, and sepsis. The overall adverse event rate is approximately 4.1 percent but varies by procedure. The open **RYGB** has a rate of 7.3 percent while the laparoscopic **RGYB** is 5.5 percent and the **LAGB** is 3 percent. These risks are low and for some are worth it to avoid the increased morbidity and mortality due to obesity.

Chapter 7

Menopause & Beyond: A New You

Once a woman has stopped having her period she is no longer able to reproduce. This is called menopause. It's a new stage of life, and while many celebrate the transition others mourn it. However, a woman feels about it, the loss of ovarian function does contribute to some health challenges while other medical conditions develop because of aging.

Menopause

"Doctor, when will this menopause thing stop? I've been having hot flashes for months now and it feels like they are getting worse. On top of this my husband is complaining because I have zero interest in sex. But tell me, who would want to have sex when it feels like pins and needles are attacking your vagina?" Sofia who is now 53 years old tells me this as soon as I walk into the consultation room.

<u>What is menopause?</u>

Menopause is defined as "the period of permanent cessation of menstruation." Culturally, however, the condition is most often discussed in the context of the perimenopausal phase. This is the transition phase when a woman's periods are becoming irregular prior to the actual permanent cessation of menses. The troublesome symptoms that accompany this transition are responsible for the infamy of this change.

Menopause results once the ovaries have stopped producing eggs. The hormonal consequence is a significant reduction in the circulating levels of estrogen, progesterone, and testosterone. For the most part, these hormones are created in the ovaries. Estrogen and testosterone can be produced in smaller quantities from other sites within the body. The average age of menopause is 51.3 years, but can range from 45 to 55 years of age.

Perimenopause is the period prior to menopause during which ovarian function is slowing and ovulation is less frequent. The menstrual cycle lengthens. This tends to occur after age 40 and can continue for 2 to 8 years before the actual menopause.

Hormone levels reflect these changes. Follicle stimulating hormone (FSH) levels tend to be increased. This hormone is working harder and harder to get the ovary to make follicles and to ovulate. The remaining follicles tend to be less responsive, so higher levels of FSH are required to stimulate them. Sometimes ovulation doesn't occur. This explains decreased fertility in this age group. The estrogen levels are not significantly reduced but may fluctuate based on the ovarian activity. At the point when there are no follicles left to respond, menstruation ceases forever!

Once the transition to menopause is complete, there may be some health consequences that can be directly associated with hormonal deficiency. Historically, estrogen has been identified as the culprit. The role of progesterone is discussed in the lay literature but has largely been unstudied despite anecdotal evidence to support its function.

The medical concerns surrounding menopause are both a result of the potential health risks and the bothersome symptoms that can interfere with quality of life. It is important to distinguish the difference.

Most of these problems are a consequence of aging, but certainly can be exacerbated by the continuing hormonal deficiency. There are other issues that are specific to hormonal deficiency. Finally, there are the annoying symptoms that are not life-threatening but can affect a person's quality of life.

Issues specific to hormone deficiency

- Vaginal Dryness
- Decreased Libido

Problems that occur with age that might be exacerbated by hormone deficiency

- Loss of bone density
- Loss of muscle mass and strength
- Hair loss
- Weight gain

Quality of life issues

- Hot flashes/night sweats
- Mood swings
- Urinary symptoms

Menopause is the post-reproductive stage of a woman's life. Because it coincides with aging there are many potential health risks that arise during this time. It is important to know your risks so you can eliminate them and develop good health habits that may counterbalance these risks.

Denise Howard, MD

Hot Flashes

"Hot flash" is the term used to describe the sudden onset of warmth or heat, which starts in the chest and spreads to the neck and face. Sweating, redness, palpitations, and anxiety usually accompany this symptom. Hot flashes are problematic because they are recurrent, happening many times in a day. Another term used to describe these events is "vasomotor symptoms." Night sweats are also part of this symptom complex. These symptoms typically are associated with menopause but can also occur in premenopausal women and women who are postpartum.

A hot flash occurs when the core body temperature suddenly increases to a level that is above a certain set threshold. Above this threshold sweating occurs and below this threshold shivering occurs. There is a temperature range that is considered to be normal when no such symptoms occur. This "neutral zone" is postulated to be much smaller in women who experience hot flashes. Thus, small changes in the core body temperature would precipitate sweating in a menopausal woman, but in a non-menopausal woman the same change would be within the neutral zone and a hot flash would not occur. The narrowing of this neutral zone is triggered by a sudden decrease in circulating estrogen levels. Estrogen and testosterone affect natural endorphins, which in turn regulate core body temperature.

Hot flashes occur in 75 percent of postmenopausal women and are the most common complaint in women transitioning to menopause. The symptoms are not life-threatening but can be distressing and disruptive. They can affect work, social interactions, and interfere with sleep. They reportedly occur 1 to 2 years before menopause and persist up to 5 years after menopause. Many women in their 40's report experiencing this phenomenon.

Women who have their ovaries surgically removed will also experience vasomotor symptoms. In many cases, they are more severe than in women who go through a natural menopause. Immediately after delivery, there is a sudden drop in circulating estrogen levels. It is therefore not surprising that postpartum women experience hot flashes as well. Women taking tamoxifen for breast cancer also suffer with vasomotor symptoms due to the anti-estrogenic effect of this drug. Men who receive certain treatments for prostate cancer that affect androgen production also experience hot flashes.

Vasomotor symptoms associated with menopause can be quite disturbing. Some women have mild symptoms or no symptoms and do not require treatment, but for others the occurrence of these flashes may be very disruptive. Hot flashes and other menopausal symptoms might become intolerable and treatment is recommended to allow normal functioning. It is important to discuss these symptoms with your doctor, who can then prescribe a treatment regimen that is right for you.

Treatment of Hot Flashes

Hot flashes are the major reason women going through the menopausal transition seek medical care. While hot flashes are not life-threatening and are not a sign of a medical disorder, they can interfere with daily functioning and quality of life, as well as cause sleep deprivation and produce anxiety. Options for treatment include hormonal and non-hormonal medication as well as behavioral therapies.

Traditional hormone replacement therapy (HRT) is the "gold standard" for treating hot flashes. It reduces hot flashes by 80 to 90 percent.[2] Hormone replacement therapy entails estrogen-only therapy in women who have undergone a hysterectomy and combined estrogen and progestin in women whose uteri are still in place. The problem with HRT is the potential risk and side effects. Side effects include weight gain, tissue swelling, breast tenderness, and uterine bleeding. Risks include blood clots in the deep veins, pulmonary embolus, heart attack, stroke, and breast cancer.

Progestin-only treatment is an option for women who can't take estrogen or who desire an estrogen-free treatment. There are many progestins on the market that decrease the incidence of hot flashes, some by 75 to 80 percent.[2] Progestin-only therapy has its problems, including symptoms of depression and possible bone loss with long-term therapy in selected products.

Tibolone is a synthetic hormone that has estrogenic, progestational, and androgenic effects. It is available in many places outside of the U.S. and is effective in the management of vasomotor symptoms. In addition to decreasing hot flashes, it also decreases vaginal dryness and some of the urinary symptoms that accompany menopause.

There are many options for managing hot flashes. Hormonal treatment is one option but many other alternatives exist. It is important to work with your health care provider to develop a plan that is right for you.

Nutritional supplements such as black cohosh, Vitamin E, and soy proteins have some reported benefits. Black cohosh is available over the counter in many pharmacies and grocery stores. Vitamin E, taken in the amount of 800 international units daily, are recommended for the management of mild hot flashes. Finally, soy extracts or increasing the amount of daily soy intake is an option for hot flash management.

Selective serotonin reuptake inhibitors have been shown to reduce flashes by 37 to 61 percent compared to a placebo.[3] These drugs are approved for the treatment of depression so they are also helpful for the mood disturbances that some women experience when going through menopause.

Gabapentin, a medication used for seizures and neuropathic pain, has been shown to decrease flashes by 46 to 49 percent.[4] The recommended dose is 900 mg a day.

Behavioral therapies include lifestyle changes that make the flashes less severe. Dressing in layers so garments can be easily removed, lowering the room temperature, and drinking cool beverages are suggested strategies. Paced respirations or slow, deep breathing can reduce flash frequency by approximately 50 percent. Stress relief and relaxation therapy are also helpful.

Hormone Replacement Therapy (HRT)

Hormone replacement therapy is the term used to describe the administration of hormones in postmenopausal women. It is an attempt to alleviate the symptoms that often occur as a result of hormone deficiency. When HRT was first introduced on the market, there was great optimism that it would have anti-aging benefits, but this was quickly dispelled when many of the negative effects came to light. Traditionally, HRT meant a combination of estrogen and progestin, but in some instances, might include testosterone.

Most HRT preparations contain a daily dose of estrogen and either a 14-day dose of progestin or a daily dose of progestin. The primary purpose of the progestin is to prevent growth of the endometrium and subsequent endometrial cancer. HRT dosage was initially designed to simulate the normal menstrual cycle. The use of a daily low-dose progestin along with estrogen was found to have a number of advantages, the most practical one being the ease of use.

After many decades of research and experience using various formulations of HRT, we have learned a lot. Currently HRT is recommended for the relief of moderate-to-severe vasomotor symptoms due to menopause. Estrogen is by far the most effective treatment for hot flashes and night sweats.

Vaginal estrogen is the first choice in the treatment of vaginal atrophy, the thinning of vaginal tissue. Previously, HRT was thought to provide some benefits in the prevention of certain chronic diseases, such as heart disease and osteoporosis. Even though there are select benefits, HRT is no longer recommended for the prevention of chronic diseases. When prescribed, it should be used for the shortest interval possible, no more than 2 to 3 years.

As with all therapies, there are some down sides. HRT is not the miracle youth pill it was initially touted to be. Estrogen alone, given to women who still have their uterus, can lead to endometrial cancer. There is now a proven association between HRT and the development of breast cancer. HRT increases the chance of venous thromboembolism (blood clots), pulmonary emboli, and stroke. In postmenopausal women, the risk of coronary heart disease is also increased. Finally, oral HRT can have an adverse effect on circulating lipid levels, which in turn increases the risk of cardiovascular disease.

Still, HRT has provided tremendous benefits for many generations of women. Menopausal symptoms can have a significant impact on the quality of life, including the family and friends of those affected. It is the duty of the health care provider to take a thorough history, perform a complete physical examination, and give in-depth counseling before prescribing HRT. Women who have a history of breast cancer, stroke, coronary heart disease, blood clots, and active liver disease should not use HRT. It is important to understand your risks and the potential benefits before starting any medications, including HRT.

Understanding HRT Preparations

There are numerous **HRT** formulations and delivery options. Progestin is typically used to prevent endometrial hyperplasia (growth of the endometrium). Most menopause-related symptoms are relieved with estrogen. The most commonly used estrogens are oral or transdermal preparations. There is an even wider variety of progestins.

HRT is typically prescribed as cyclic or continuous. Cyclic regimens tend to have 21 to 28 days of estrogen and then 14 days of progestin. Consequently, many women will experience a withdrawal bleed like a normal menses. Continuous HRT has a daily low dose of progestin, designed to prevent the growth of the endometrium and thus eliminating the cyclic withdrawal bleeding that is mostly unwelcome.

There are a variety of **HRT** delivery routes. Formulations are designed to be used orally, transdermally, and by transvaginal routes. The preparations have evolved over time but tend to include pills, patches, mists, sprays, gels, lotions, implants, strings, and rings. Alternate routes of **HRT** administration were developed in response to the notorious "first-pass effect" of oral estrogen (it passed through liver before going to the rest of the body). When taken by mouth, estrogen can build up in the liver, with high concentrations leading to increased production of substances such as lipids, clotting factors, and binding globulins. This increased production leads to an increased risk of blood clots and increased circulating lipid levels, which contribute to increased risk of cardiovascular disease. Delivery via other routes eliminates this "first past effect," resulting in a lower risk of these problems.

The term "bioidentical hormones" has been introduced into the discussion of HRT, and for many it translates into a safer or better product. However, the term tends to be used interchangeably with "natural" hormones or compounded hormones. For many, natural means it is derived from plants. Equine estrogen is natural because it is derived from animals and not synthesized in a manufacturing plant. Many women, however, object to the use of horse-derived estrogens. "Compounded" simply means that the batch of medication is made on demand rather than having a pre-made formulation. The advantage to compounding is that the dosage can be tailored to individual demand. "Bio-identical" means the medication is structurally identical to the hormones people produce themselves. Many of the pre-made synthetic formulations, such as estradiol and prometrium, are bio-identical. So, in fact, conjugated equine estrogen is a natural product but not bio-identical.

Prescribing HRT is not a simple endeavor. If you think you may need hormone replacement therapy it is important that you consult with an experienced clinician. The first step is assessing your need and your risks, and the second is selecting the combination and type of therapy that best suits you.

Benefits of HRT

In addition to all the positive effects estrogen has on the reproductive system, it also has a positive effect on other parts of the body, including bones. The presence of estrogen helps to maintain bone density. Once a woman goes through menopause, she has a significant reduction in bone density, which then places her at higher risk of osteoporosis and related fractures. Women on estrogen have a much lower risk of osteoporotic and related bone fractures, and even though estrogen replacement should not be the first line therapy for osteoporosis prevention it should certainly be considered in many cases.

There are other notable benefits of estrogen replacement. Women on HRT have a much lower risk of developing type 2 diabetes mellitus. This is thought to be due to the favorable effect on insulin utilization.

There is less insulin resistance in those on HRT. Women taking HRT are also less likely to develop colorectal cancer. Finally, menopausal women can develop recurrent urinary tract infections due to the effects of urogenital atrophy. Local estrogen therapy reduces this risk.

The general recommendations for HRT is that it should be utilized in symptomatic women, at the lowest effective dose and for the shortest period possible, and for no longer than 5 years. Individualization of treatment can be made for those who have no other risks as longer-term treatment can be an option for them.

Risks of HRT

In women who have had their uterus surgically removed, there isn't a need for progestin, so estrogen replacement therapy (ERT) is prescribed. All medications and therapies have their potential risks and it is important to understand these before accepting any treatment.

HRT has experienced a pendulum-like effect in its popularity. When first introduced, ERT was thought to be a wonder drug and then the association with endometrial cancer was recognized. The addition of progestin to the regimen minimized this risk and it was again very popular. Recent studies have shown an association with breast cancer and an increased risk of other conditions resulting in a more conservative approach to the prescribing of this treatment.

The absolute risk of HRT in women in their 50s with use for less than 5 years is low, and those who have been menopausal for more than 10 years or are in their 60s are at greater risk. The increased risks noted here involve the use of HRT for more than 5 years.

Breast cancer is the most common cancer in women, and the news that HRT increased this risk was the most shocking revelation of recent large studies. The risk was increased by 6.8 additional cases per 1,000 women after more than 5 years of use of combined estrogen and progestin therapy. This risk was not increased in those women using estrogen alone.[6]

HRT also increases the risk of thromboembolic events (blood clots), a fact known from the birth control pill experience. The overall risk of venous thromboembolism is 2 to 5 cases per 1000 women and 1 to 1.2 cases of stroke. Women taking combination therapy had an increased risk of coronary heart disease at 8 additional cases per 10,000 person years. The risk was not increased in those taking estrogen alone or in those under 59 years of age.[7]

HRT also has an undesirable effect on the cholesterol and triglyceride levels. The increase in lipids most likely contributes to an increased risk of heart disease and blood clots. This effect is much less with transdermal administration.

Hormone replacement therapy in certain combinations and preparations increases the risk of breast cancer, heart disease, and blood clots.

No therapy is without its risks and it is therefore important to weigh the benefits against the risks when selecting any treatment. HRT has provided benefit to generations of women and even though there are some untoward effects, it is a viable option in women who are at low risk of complications.

THE BOTTOM LINE

- Every woman will experience menopause.
- Most of the bothersome symptoms occur because of low estrogen.
- There are pros and cons to using hormone replacement therapy.

Bone Health

Liz came to see me for a routine examination. In taking her history I learn that she had her ovaries removed at age 32 for severe endometriosis. At age 54 she is trying to remain active and had started training for a triathlon. "My back hurts all the time," she declares when I asked her how she felt. After completing the physical examination, I told Liz that I wanted to order a bone density scan. I explained that I was concerned about her bones because she had premature menopause due to the surgical removal of her ovaries and that with her small stature she was at risk of osteoporosis.

What is osteoporosis?

Osteoporosis is a disorder of the skeletal system that results in decreased bone strength and subsequent susceptibility to fractures. It is a major epidemiologic (affects a large number of the population) problem and the prevalence is rapidly increasing due to an aging population. Osteoporotic bones are easily fractured and even a minimal impact could cause breakage. The hip and spine are the areas most commonly affected. Hip fractures are common reasons older individuals lose their independence, and can even lead to death if not treated quickly. It is important to understand normal bone structure and the abnormalities that lead to this disorder in order to understand prevention and treatment.

Bone strength is determined by bone density and bone quality. Components of this are structural and material in nature. Structural properties include bone shape, size, and microarchitecture (their internal structure). Material properties include mineralization, collagen composition, and damage accumulation.

Bone mineral density testing is the standard way to measure bone integrity. This testing is performed using dual-energy x-ray absorptiometry (DEXA). The World Health Organization (WHO) has defined criteria for normal and abnormal results. The T score is utilized and describes the number of standard deviations (SD) in which a person's results exceeds (positive score) or falls below (negative score) the mean of a young adult group of the same sex.

Osteoporosis is the diagnosis when the value falls 2.5 standard deviations (T score of −2.5) or more below the mean. Osteopenia or low bone density occurs when the T score is −1.0 to −2.5. If the score is greater than −1.0, one's bones are of normal density. These ranges were developed to identify individuals who are at increased risk of fractures. The goal of early diagnosis and prevention is to minimize the incidence of fracture and other morbidity as they can have life-threatening and life-altering consequences.

How does it occur?

Osteoporosis occurs when the bone density falls to a point that there is an increased risk of fracture with minimal trauma. The risk of developing osteoporosis is determined by the peak bone density achieved during childhood and the rate of bone loss later in life. Bone strength is due to the density of the bone, but also bone quality. Bone density is easier to measure and therefore discussed more. In order to understand osteoporosis, it is first important to understand how normal bone is maintained.

Healthy bone is maintained by a balance between the destruction of old, damaged bone and the formation of new bone. Cells called "osteoclasts" remove old bone by producing substances that destroy the old bone. Cells called "osteoblasts" secrete new bone material into the cavity where the old bone was removed. This process of bone resorption and formation, called remodeling, is how a skeleton maintains its strength.

An individual continues to build bone during childhood and adulthood. The maximum achieved bone mass is complete by age 40, however childhood bone development is the most crucial. The peak bone mass achieved is determined by environmental and genetic factors.

Bone loss occurs because of an imbalance between the activity of the osteoclasts and osteoblasts. Postmenopausal women develop significantly increased bone turnover, which continues for many years after the cessation of ovarian function. This is due to a decrease in estrogen production. This loss of estrogen leads to an increase in the life span of the osteoclasts (cells that destroy bone) and a shortening of the life span of the osteoblasts (cells that make new bone).

Understanding how bone works leads to a better understanding of risk factors for developing low bone density and osteoporosis. Menopause and early menopause are major risk factors due to the increased bone turnover that occurs once estrogen production stops.

Caucasian women are at increased risk because of a lower peak bone mass achieved when compared to women of other racial groups. Smoking and excessive alcohol use can also lead to increased bone loss. Other factors that contribute to an increased risk of osteoporosis include certain medications, specific medical conditions, Vitamin D deficiency, and poor calcium absorption.

Knowing the risks for osteoporosis is helpful in targeting prevention and early diagnosis. The overall goal is fracture prevention, which is the cause of excessive morbidity and mortality. Current options for prevention and treatment are effective but there are many people who are unaware of their risks and many healthcare providers who do not discuss this problem. As with many disorders, prevention and early intervention is the key to minimize poor outcomes.

<u>Why is it a problem?</u>

The annual direct cost of osteoporotic related fractures is estimated to be $17 to $20 billion in the U.S. and $30 billion in the European Union. The cost is estimated to be $50 billion in the U.S. by 2040. The costs are greater than the health care costs of breast cancer, stroke, and diabetes.

Approximately 8 million women in the United States and 200 million worldwide have osteoporosis. Twenty-two million people in the U.S. have low bone mineral density. It is estimated that by 2020, 14 million people in the U.S. over the age of 50 will suffer from this condition. Women are at greater risk than men. Race also plays a role. The table below summarizes the percentage of women by racial group over age 50 that are affected.[11]

	Osteoporosis	Low bone mineral density
White, Asian	22%	52%
Black	5%	35%
Hispanic	10%	49%

Even though Asian people tend to have lower bone density, their risk of developing a fracture is no greater than for black or Hispanic people. Even though black people are less likely to experience fractures, they are at greater risk of disability and death if they do experience a hip fracture.

Hip fractures are the most devastating consequence of osteoporosis and typically occur after a fall. The estimates for this are expected to reach 6.3 million by 2050. Twenty percent of people who experience a hip fracture die within a year of the event; 33 percent require nursing home placement, and less than 33 percent regain their previous level of physical fitness. Fractures can occur in other areas too, such as the spine. This can result in loss of height and chronic back pain. Of the people who experience fractures that are obviously due to fragile bones, less than 25 percent are evaluated for osteoporosis.

Given the economic burden and risks of disability and mortality it is imperative that everyone become aware of this treatable and preventable disorder.

Who is at risk?

Fifteen percent of women will develop a hip fracture by age 80. Once a woman develops one fracture, she is at greater risk of developing a second. One study showed that those with a vertebral fracture have a 19 percent chance of developing a second fracture within 1 year. All of this is due to osteoporosis.

Identifying women who are at risk is important so that preventative measures and early treatment can be undertaken. The overall goal is the prevention of fractures. The following are common factors that are associated with the development of osteoporosis and related fractures:

- Postmenopausal women
- Early menopause
- Poor calcium absorption
- Low body weight
- Steroid use
- Smoking
- Certain medical disorders
- Certain medications
- Vitamin D deficiency
- History of fractures
- Family history of fractures
- Excessive alcohol consumption

There are simple strategies that can be adopted by anyone to prevent the development of this problem and related fractures:

- Increase calcium and Vitamin D in your diet or via supplements—1200 mg of calcium and 400-800 international units of Vitamin D.
- Muscle Strengthening: weight bearing, aerobic, strength training, and stretching. Protects against osteoporosis, fractures, and falls. Improves flexibility and balance.
- Fall prevention in those at risk: dizziness, poor vision, decreased mobility, poor muscle strength and coordination, and urinary incontinence.
- Smoking cessation.
- Moderate alcohol consumption.

Osteoporosis is preventable and treatable. All women and children should get adequate calcium and Vitamin D in their diet. Regular exercise 3 to 4 times per week for at least 30 minutes has been proven to be effective in maintaining bone density and even reversing bone loss. The other benefits are improved coordination and increased muscle strength, minimizing the risks of falls.

Diagnostic tools should be utilized for those at risk, allowing for early diagnosis and appropriate intervention. All women who have risk factors or who are over age 65 should undergo bone density testing.

Medications for Osteoporosis Prevention and Treatment

There are many medications available for the prevention and treatment of osteoporosis. They improve bone mineral density and have been proven to significantly decrease the risk of fractures. The currently available medications are listed below.

Estrogen in the form of traditional hormone replacement therapy has been proven to improve bone density and reduce the risk of fractures of the hip, spine (vertebral), and wrist. It acts by preventing bone resorption by inhibiting osteoclast formation and function. It also prolongs the life span of the osteoblast.

The concerns of hormone therapy are the small association with the diagnosis of breast cancer and the increased risk of thromboembolic events such as blood clots and stroke. At this point, there are other effective medications and therefore estrogen would not be recommended as a first-line therapy for osteoporosis.

Studies have documented increased bone loss after discontinuation of estrogen. All women who elect to stop hormone therapy should be assessed for the risk of osteoporosis and treated appropriately.

Biphosphonates include a group of medications that act by destroying the osteoclasts. The result is a significant decrease in bone turnover and bone loss. These medications have been proven thus far to be the most effective in fracture reduction. Studies have documented a 40 to 50 percent reduction in vertebral fractures and a 20 to 40 percent reduction in non-vertebral fractures, including hip fractures.

They include alendronate, risedronate, ibandronate and zoledronic acid. Therapies include daily, weekly, monthly, quarterly, and yearly regimens.

Side effects can include gastrointestinal problems such as ulcers and abdominal pain. In addition, there is a rare occurrence of necrosis of the jawbone. Also, if you stop using the medication you could experience increased bone turnover and a decrease in bone density, meaning a higher risk of fractures.

Selective estrogen receptor modulators (SERMS) exert estrogen-like effects on selective tissues while avoiding some of the undesired effects of estrogen. Raloxifene, the SERM that has been studied in osteoporosis, acts by decreasing bone turnover and has been proven to decrease the risk of vertebral fractures by 34 to 50 percent. Its side effects include hot flashes and an increased risk of thromboembolic events. The potential benefit is that it has demonstrated effectiveness in breast cancer prevention and may soon be approved for this use.

Calcitonin inhibits osteoclast activity to prevent bone resorption. It is available in an injectable form and as a nasal spray. It has been shown to decrease the risk of spinal fractures in people with osteoporosis by 33 percent. It is generally well tolerated.

Parathyroid hormone is available as a daily subcutaneous injection called Teriparatide. The exact mechanism of action is unclear; however, it appears to stimulate bone formation even on inactive bone surfaces. The activity of both the osteoclast and osteob-last is increased, with an overall net effect of increased bone formation. Studies have demonstrated an increase in bone density of both the hip and spine. They also report a 69 percent reduction in spinal fractures and a 53 percent reduction in non-vertebral fractures. Adverse effects include nausea, headaches, and an increase in serum calcium levels. There was also an observed increase in the incidence of osteosarcoma (bone cancer) in animal studies. For this reason, it is only recommended for cases of severe osteoporosis and those at high risk of fracture. This medication should not be used for longer than 2 years. The benefits in terms of improved bone density will disappear when the medication is stopped, so using another agent is advised after discontinuation.

There are many effective medications available for the prevention and treatment of osteoporosis. In cases of severe disease there is also the option of combination treatment with 2 agents that have different mechanisms of action. No medication is completely free of risk or side effects, but you can work closely with your health care provider to choose the one that is right for you.

There are other relatively new medications on the market that have the potential to be effective alternatives. Denosumab is a monoclonal antibody that decreases osteoclastic activity. It was approved by the FDA for the treatment of postmenopausal osteoporosis. Tibolone, a synthetic steroid whose metabolites have estrogenic, progesteronic, and androgenic properties, has been shown to increase bone mineral density, prevent bone loss, and decrease fractures. Unfortunately, it is not currently available in the U.S.

THE BOTTOM LINE

- Osteoporosis is a condition of thin bones.
- The concern about Osteoporosis relates to the ease in which the bones can be broken.
- There are many things that can be done to keep your bones strong.

Vulvar Disorders

"Listen doc, I'm itching down there all the time and its driving me crazy. I know it can't be a STD because I haven't been intimate in years." Mikayla explains to me when I ask the reason for her visit. At 75 years old, she is highly distressed that she is experiencing problems with her genital area and needs some help. "I've been to five different doctors and none of them knows what's going on."

Understanding Vulvar Disorders

Vulvar symptoms such as itching, pain, lesions, or growths can result from a variety of disorders. Any problem that occurs in the skin can present in the vulvar area. There are also certain conditions that are specific to this anatomical region by virtue of the tissue composition at this site.

The female genital region includes the labia minora, labia majora, the clitoris, urethra and the entrance to the birth canal also referred to as the introitus. The tissue in this area is composed of skin, mucous membrane, glands, and hair bearing structures. Abnormalities can occur in any of these areas. The problems that arise can be due to infection, inflammation, or as a result of a benign or malignant process.

The most common symptom is itching which is typically the first sign of a yeast (candida) infection. Other infectious processes include folliculitis, which arises from the hair follicles, herpes simplex infection, which has other characteristic features, and syphilis, which also has other classic findings.

Cancer can certainly occur in the vulvar area but is quite rare. This is, however, the greatest concern whenever an unexplained, persistent problem occurs. Early diagnosis is paramount since treatment is possible when cancer is found at an early stage. Vulvar cancer should be suspected if there is an ulcer that does not heal or a mass that is fleshy and bleeds easily. Other concerning signs are hard nodules, a warty looking growth and a single lesion especially in postmenopausal women.

Other signs of malignancy include lesions which are asymmetric, have irregular borders and color variation. A rapidly changing lesion, one that bleeds and does not heal, is also highly suspicious for cancer. A biopsy should be taken of any area of concern. This is easily performed in the outpatient setting with a local anesthetic.

Vulvar Growths

Genital warts will commonly present as a new growth in the vulva area. Their appearance may vary but typically look like miniature cauliflower. These are caused by infection with human papilloma virus. Types 6 and 11 cause over 90 percent of genital warts. They generally resolve over time however their appearance and discomfort sometimes lead women to seek care. They can also lead to vulvar cancer in rare cases. The warts can be treated in several ways. They can be excised or treated with a local acid solution, however this must be done by a doctor. Podophyllin and imiquimod cream can be prescribed for home use.

Another infectious related skin problem is molluscum contagiosum. It is caused by a pox virus and is more common in immunosuppressed individuals. It presents with scattered pearly or translucent papules with an umbilicated center. The treatment is the same as for genital warts.

Acrochordon or skin tags are commonly found in the vulvar area and inner thigh. They are pedunculated soft fibromas, which tend to develop in areas of friction. Therefore, are more common in obese or overweight women. They can be excised in the office with a local anesthetic.

Cysts are fluid filled structures, which are usually benign. Sebaceous or epidermal cyst can occur in the skin of the vulva. These cysts can occur anywhere on the skin and result when the skin cells become trapped beneath the surface and the exfoliated cells and glandular material build up creating a cystic structure. These cysts can sometimes become infected and may need to be excised if they get too large.

The Bartholin's gland secretes fluid that helps lubricate the birth canal. It is located just inside the introitus at the entrance to the birth canal. If the duct becomes obstructed this fluid has nowhere to drain and tends to build up, causing a Bartholin's cyst. If this cyst gets infected, then it is known as an abscess. Bartholin's abscess presents with pain and swelling in the genital area. In many cases, it may rupture spontaneously providing immediate relief or may require incision and drainage by a health care provider.

There are also many other unusual growths that can appear in the vulvar area. Examples are lipomas, which are fatty tumors, leiomyomas which are tumors of the smooth cells and fibromas. These tend to be benign but in rare cases can be malignant. Even hernias can present with growths in the vulvar area.

Vulvar growths can result from any number of causes. The vast majority are benign and can be managed easily. If you have an unusual growth it is best to see your gynecologist who can help determine the source of the problem.

Vulvar Plaques and Patches

The vulvar skin, like the rest of the body, can develop allergic reactions and autoimmune responses that cause unusual patches, or "plaques." The appearance and other associated symptoms can help determine the cause of these skin changes. The symptoms may include itching or irritation, pain or discomfort, and flaking skin. On examination, the doctor may find changes in the skin texture, erosions, white patches, and areas of redness. A biopsy may be required to determine the problem; however, an experienced gynecologist may be able to diagnose the problem just by looking. The disorders below are some of the more common causes of plaques and patches.

Lichen Simplex Chronicus

This is essentially a dermatitis (inflammation of the skin) that has developed from chronic scratching or rubbing, possibly as a result of a yeast infection or an allergic reaction to a chemical. The itch/scratch cycle is a vicious one that is difficult to break. The more you scratch, the more you itch, and it is the scratching that leads to the chronic problem.

On examination, the skin will appear thickened, flaky, and may have white or dark patches depending on the natural skin color. There may be erosions or excoriations (sores or lesions) from scratching. Breaking the cycle can solve the problem. Treatment may include local medication to stop the itching and oral medication to decrease the inflammatory reaction. Topical steroid ointment and oral antihistamine medications are the most commonly used. Other recommendations may include cutting your nails or wearing gloves at nighttime to minimize the trauma of scratching during sleep.

Lichen Sclerosus

This is a condition in which the skin of the vulva is essentially destroyed. The cause is unknown. It presents with itching or irritation that gradually worsens over years and can lead to pain with intercourse. On examination, the skin is noted to be thin, wrinkled, and white. The classic description is that it looks like cigarette paper.

Over time the changes can lead to destruction of the normal anatomy. The labia may shrink and disappear and the clitoris may become buried under scar tissue. Minimal trauma can cause tearing.

The goal of treatment is to prevent further damage. The doctor will prescribe a high-potency steroid ointment to apply to the skin. Continued monitoring by an experienced gynecologist or dermatologist is required because women with this condition are at a higher risk of developing vulvar cancer.

<u>Vitiligo</u>

Vitiligo is an autoimmune skin condition that can affect the whole body. The cells that produce skin color are called melanocytes. When they are destroyed, or are not functioning properly, there is a lack of skin color that usually looks like a notable, well-defined white patch. The skin is otherwise healthy in appearance. The absence of other symptoms and the findings of white patches in other body areas is an indication that the condition is vitiligo. The treatment is best managed by a dermatologist.

<u>Other Causes</u>

Other causes of patches and plaques include skin lesions that can be found in other parts of the body. Nevi and moles are common, as well as dermatitis, psoriasis, and seborrheic keratosis, which occur with age. These dermatologic problems tend to be benign, but you should always be concerned about lesions that change appearance rapidly, bleed easily, have irregular borders, or are black in color. It is important to see a gynecologist or dermatologist immediately if you have any concerns.

THE BOTTOM LINE

- Vulvar problems can sometimes be difficult to diagnose.
- Keep a record of all treatments prescribed and how long you used them. This will help your doctor in determining the best approach.
- If you are experiencing problems and your gynecologist hasn't been able to help, ask for a referral to a Gynecologist or Dermatologist who has a special interest in Vulvar disorders.

Chapter 8

The Things You Can Do Something About!

A part of living is dying, and we all will die of something, but what we all hope, pray, and desire is to live a long and prosperous life. Unfortunately, there are some life-threatening events that can't be prevented or predicted. However, there are many measures we can take to minimize the risks of these incidents. A great example is wearing seat belts. We all recognize that when we travel in a motor vehicle, especially in heavy traffic, there is a chance of having an accident. According to the National Highway Traffic Safety Administration, wearing seat belts reduces the risk of death or injury by approximately 50 percent.[1] This simple measure improves your chances of surviving, even if the accident is serious.

There are many potential steps you can take to decrease your chance of poor health. If you consistently eat a healthy diet, exercise on a regular basis, avoid the overuse of substances, and take advantage of the preventative health tests discussed earlier in this book, then the probability is high that you will live your full life expectancy.

The goal of this chapter is to provide you with the basic information you need to make the right choices about diet, exercise, and substance use.

Nutrition

The first step to ensuring good health is to consume a healthy diet. Your body needs fuel to function. Every food has a specific energy source and contains other nutrients to maximize ideal function. This section will discuss nutrition, the components of a proper diet, the nutrients contained within food, and how our body utilizes the food consumed.

Nutrition versus Diet

Our society is conflicted! We want fast food and great looking bodies. We place higher value on athletic physiques but eat for entertainment and groan if we have to walk up a few flights of stairs. This incongruity has led to a societal obsession with nutrition and dieting.

Nutrition is the study of food at work in our bodies, our source of energy, and the medium for which our nutrients can function. Nutrition is the building block of life and is just one key to developing and maintaining good health. Nutrition encompasses a whole range of areas, including the utilization of food so the body can remain healthy, grow, repair and maintain its function. It deals with getting the proper amounts of nutrients from food and making smart food choices.

Diet typically refers to a food regimen designed to achieve a goal such as losing weight. However, diet really describes the food we eat in the course of a time period such as 24-hours, one week, or one month. From a health perspective, an ideal diet is a nutritional lifestyle that promotes good health. It must include several food groups because a single group cannot provide all the nutrients humans need for good health.

The CDC estimates that up to 40 percent of deaths from the top 5 leading causes are potentially preventable. These top 5 causes include heart disease, cancer, and stroke, which in many cases result from poor nutrition and other lifestyle choices. Nutrition is important because it is the foundation of a productive, healthy life. This foundation starts while you are still *in utero*, with the habits of your mother, and continue through infancy, childhood, adolescence, young adulthood, and the rest of your life. That's why it's important to start making wise choices about diet and lifestyle as early as possible.

Each developmental period has different energy and nutritional requirements. In addition, other lifestyle choices and health challenges may affect these nutritional needs. It is important to develop an understanding of proper nutrition and its components, but also to recognize that individual needs will change over time and be prepared to adjust your diet to address these needs. The goal is to give your body exactly what it needs to meet the demands of life; more or less may contribute to the development of health issues over time. Remember the goal of good nutrition is to maintain a healthy body so you can function at the highest level possible.

Digestion

Our body requires essential nutrients to function. We acquire our energy through the consumption of food, which is then gradually broken down to the molecular level to be absorbed by the cells in our body. The process by which food is converted into energy is complex and fascinating, but it all starts with digestion.

The digestive system is the body's organ system responsible for digestion, absorption, and defecation. It includes the gastrointestinal tract, as well as the organs that produce and store the chemicals needed in digestion. The gastrointestinal tract includes the mouth, esophagus, stomach, small intestine and the large intestine. The liver and pancreas produce chemicals that help break down food for absorption. The gall bladder stores bile, which is produced in the liver.

The small intestine includes the duodenum, jejunum, and the ileum. The large intestine is also called the colon, and includes the right, left, and transverse colon. The first part of the colon, the cecum, is located on the right-hand side of the body and is also the location of the appendix. The colon terminates on the left side with the sigmoid, which transitions to become the rectum. Finally, there is the anus, which is the exit from the body.

Digestion starts in the mouth, with the chewing, or "mastication," of food. Chewing builds up saliva, which contains enzymes that aid in the breakdown of food. When food is thoroughly chewed, and mixed with saliva it's called a bolus, which is what you swallow when you're eating. The bolus is transported to the stomach through the esophagus. It remains in the stomach for 1 to 2 hours, where gastric juices and stomach peristalsis—the muscles contracting and squeezing—continue the process of breaking down the food into a mixture called "chime." From here it enters the duodenum and then passes through the rest of the small intestine.

In the small intestine, food is further mixed with chemicals and hormones from the pancreas and liver. At this stage the food is broken down into nutrients, which can be absorbed into the blood. The remaining substance is transported to the large intestine, where undigested carbohydrates are further broken down. This is done by bacteria in the colon, through a process called fermentation. The last of the re-absorption of water and minerals occurs in the colon, and the leftover product waste is the feces that gets expelled through the anus via a process called defecation.

The small intestine is responsible for the absorption of the bulk of the nutrients. It reabsorbs the water and minerals, preventing dehydration. The process of fermentation creates gas in the intestine, and when a large amount of undigested carbohydrates arrives in the colon the result is excessive flatulence (gassiness) and bloating. This occurs in individuals who may have a deficiency in certain digestive enzymes, such as lactase, which helps break down dairy products.

The process of digestion is important in maintaining normal body function, but problems can occur in any step in the process, contributing to problems such as heartburn, ulcers, diarrhea, pain, flatulence, malabsorption, and nutritional deficiencies.

Essential Nutrients

The crucial part of healthy eating is a balanced diet. A good diet is a balanced diet, and that means consuming from the different food groups in the right quantities. Nutritionists say there are five main food groups—grains, fruits, vegetables, protein (lean meat, poultry, beans, eggs, fish, nuts etc.), and dairy products—which supply the body with what it needs to remain healthy. Fat, sugar, and water are sometimes described as food groups, however the first two components are readily contained within the 5 major groups and water is a different focus. These major groups provide the essential nutrients the body needs to function.

Macronutrients are the structural and energy-giving caloric components of our foods that most of us are familiar with. These are the compounds consumed in large quantities, which provide the bulk of our energy. They include carbohydrates, fats, and proteins. Fiber is also a macronutrient, but serves a different function than providing energy. The U.S dietary guidelines recommend a balanced daily diet consisting of 45 to 65 percent carbohydrates, 10 to 35 percent protein, 20 to 35 percent fat and 25 to 35 grams of fiber. This is a general guideline and should be adjusted depending on an individual's body type, health, and fitness goals.

Protein, carbohydrates, and fats are our energy nutrients; they contain the fuel our bodies need to function effectively. We burn calories all the time, like a car burns gasoline to run. Our bodies need energy for every function from the beating of the heart, to brain processing, talking, walking and, of course, exercising. Without an energy source, we would wither and die quickly.

Micronutrients are those food components that are needed in small amounts to support the body's functions. These include vitamins and minerals, whose presence is needed in just the right amount; too much or too little can lead to problems. For instance, excessive amounts of sodium can contribute to hypertension while a low amount of Vitamin D and calcium may cause problems with the bones.

Vitamins and minerals are required as micro–building blocks to maintain a strong and healthy body. We can survive a long time with a deficiency in micronutrients, but like water eating away at a rock, the effects will be seen over time. We are just realizing the roles micronutrients play in preventing chronic problems such as heart disease, cancer, and diabetes. Macro and micronutrients are not only the foundation for a strong body, but also one that functions well over the long haul. Remember, the goal of good nutrition is to maintain a healthy body so you can function at the highest level possible.

What are calories?

Sometimes it seems like everyone is trying to lose weight, and all of them are trying one type of popular diet or another. The number of calories consumed and burned is a topic of conversation bordering on obsession. But what is a calorie?

A calorie is simply a way of measuring the amount of energy we use. One calorie represents the amount of heat energy it takes to raise the temperature of 1 gram of water by 1 degree Celsius. A kilocalorie represents 1,000 calories. This is often written as Calorie, which is the same as a kilocalorie.

We burn calories all the time to keep our bodies functioning and healthy. A typical adult can burn 1,500 to 2,500 calories per day to fuel their normal activities. Generally, women need fewer calories and men need more. Calorie requirements vary depending on an individual's body type, activity level, age, and overall health. Competitive athletes burn significantly more while someone who sits all day may burn much fewer than average. Growing children have a higher daily caloric requirement than a fully-grown adult. Pregnant women require more because they are providing the fuel for themselves and a developing fetus.

All nutritious calories come from carbohydrates, fat, and protein. This is why they are called the energy nutrients. Carbohydrates and protein provide 4 calories per gram while fat provides 9 calories per gram. In situations where food sources are limited, fat is a highly desired sustenance because it provides more than twice the amount of energy as an equivalent amount of protein or carbohydrate. Alcohol contains 7 calories per gram, but is not a recommended fuel for the human body.

The daily energy used can come from the calories just consumed or can be pulled from stored calories. The body stores calories in several ways. Carbohydrates are either immediately available in the blood stream as glucose, which was recently absorbed, or as glycogen, which is stored in the liver and muscle fibers.

The body stores about 2,000 calories as carbohydrates. Fat is stored intramuscularly or as adipose tissue beneath the skin and around the internal organs. There are approximately 50 to 100,000 calories stored as fat in the average body composed of 10 to 30 percent fat. Protein, which should not be used as a sole energy source, is stored in the muscles of our body. There are up to 30,000 calories stored within muscles. They are utilized in a small percentage during endurance exercises or in individuals who are malnourished, especially those who have had a long illness.

A good understanding of calories and how they are used is required when you are attempting to meet your weight management goals. This information helps you to make better food choices to meet your nutritional needs, which will vary depending on whether you are over- or underweight, undergoing medical therapy, or undertaking a physically demanding challenge.

How the Body Uses Nutrients

Food is the body's energy source. It is the fuel we need to function. Without it we cannot move, think, see, talk, grow, or reproduce. The body will either use its daily intake of fuel immediately or store it for future use. The body is quite efficient at utilizing what we give it through a variety of processes.

The main fuels for the body are carbohydrates, fat, and protein. These nutrients are provided through a variety of food sources. Once consumed, the nutrients are digested by the gastrointestinal system and taken up into the blood stream, then directed to the tissues for uptake by individual cells.

Carbohydrates are the most efficient energy source. They are converted into glucose during the digestive process and with the assistance of insulin are used immediately. Carbohydrates are the preferred food for the brain, and when not utilized are stored in the liver as glycogen. The body stores enough glucose for 1 to 2 days' use. Additional glucose can be converted to fat for long-term storage in adipose tissue.

Fats are converted into fatty acids when digested. These fatty acids are used for the maintenance and health of the body and are involved in a number of functions, such as absorption of certain vitamins, brain development, and the production of cells. Fat is stored in cells called adipocytes, and this makes up the adipose or fat tissue. This tissue insulates the body and provides it with fuel when glucose is not available.

Protein is converted to amino acids when digested. This is the material needed to develop muscles and hormones, to heal and repair. Protein can also be converted into glucose and stored as fat when the body does not immediately utilize it.

Glucose is utilized for energy by the body. It is either taken directly from a recently digested meal or from glycogen, which is stored in the liver. Once this source is used up, the body taps into its fat storage. An individual with up to 30 percent body fat has enough energy stored for over 40 days use. During periods of starvation, when fat is no longer available, non-essential proteins, such as those found in muscle, are utilized for energy. Death is imminent when essential proteins are a body's only remaining source of energy.

Understanding how the body utilizes nutrients is important in planning your diet, which must contain the right balance of carbohydrates, protein, and fats to meet your nutritional needs and to reach your health goals. Weight loss, weight gain, competitive athletics, outdoor adventures, pregnancy, and other physical states have unique nutritional requirements. To achieve the best possible outcome, you must provide your body with the appropriate fuel. Remember, the goal of good nutrition is to maintain a healthy body so you can function at the highest level possible. In the case of pregnancy, it also gives the child their best health "head start."

What are proteins?

Protein is one of the macronutrients and one of the 3 major sources of fuel for our bodies. Protein is obtained from a variety of sources and used in a number of ways by our bodies to build muscle, help with cellular function, and to store energy. This section will review the way the body uses protein to function.

Proteins are often referred to as the building blocks of the body. This is because our muscles are made up of tiny strands of protein called amino acids, which give the body its basic shape and support. We are constantly breaking down these strands, so they must be continually replaced. Protein's other vital roles include maintaining healthy skin, hair, and nails; producing hormones; aiding in sexual development; and sustaining healthy levels of red blood cells (which carry oxygen through the body). Although it is the second most plentiful substance in the body, after water, it is also the energy nutrient we need to consume the least. As with fat, it's the quality of the protein we eat that determines our health. Most people eat enough calories per day to satisfy the body's daily requirements. In fact, we will usually take in more than we actually need and this is converted to fat for storage.

There are 20 different amino acids in the body's protein. The body is able to manufacture some of these itself, but there are eight essential amino acids that cannot be made by the body and must be consumed. A deficiency of even one of these eight can lead to problems with the production of protein structures.

Foods that are rich in protein do not always contain all the essential amino acids. If the food contains all eight, it is termed complete; foods that are low in one or more are termed incomplete. Most meats and dairy products are complete protein foods, while most vegetables and fruits are incomplete. Ideally, we should eat a mixture of animal and vegetable sources to ensure that we are getting the full complement.

It is possible to get all the required amino acids from fruits and vegetables, but foods must be carefully selected. Vegetarians should take care to include beans or peas in at least two of their meals each day. They should also combine incomplete proteins, such as grains (cereals, pasta and breads), with milk or milk products (such as cheese and yogurt). Grains can be combined with legumes to achieve the same effect, and seeds can also be a good source of protein if combined with legumes. The proteins that can be obtained from vegetable sources are not as easily absorbed as those from meat sources. Vitamin C can aid this process, so vegetarians should eat or drink foods rich in this vitamin with their meals. Good sources of vitamin C include oranges and orange juice.

High quality sources of protein are essential to maintain a healthy body and mind. The body can produce most of the amino acids it needs to build muscle and maintain other functions; however, the essential amino acids must be obtained from food. The ideal sources are meat and dairy products, but careful selection of other sources can provide the body with what it needs. If you are experiencing muscle wasting, fatigue, a change in skin or hair texture, weakness, and poor immune response, you might want to examine your protein intake.

What are carbohydrates?

Dr. David Jenkins created the glycemic index (GI) to learn which foods are best for people with diabetes. The glycemic index helps you compare the quality of carbohydrates in different foods. Instead of categorizing carbohydrates as simple or complex, the GI ranks foods using a scale ranging from 0 to 100, 100 being the value assigned to the absorption of an equivalent amount of pure glucose. Foods that quickly raise the blood glucose levels receive a higher glycemic index number than foods that raise blood glucose levels more slowly.

Low GI foods have values of 55 or less. They include pumpernickel, stone ground whole wheat, rolled or steel cut oatmeal, bran, mueslix, sweet potatoes, legumes, lentils, and most fruits, among others.

Medium GI foods have values of 56 to 79 and include whole wheat, rye, quick oats, wild or basmati rice, and couscous. High glycemic foods have an index above 70 and include white breads, most cold cereals, instant oatmeal, rice, pasta, short grain rice, melons, pineapple, and crackers. Refined foods tend to have a higher glycemic index while those foods that have minimal refinement will have a lower GI. An example is steel cut oatmeal versus quick oats versus instant oatmeal.

Your body responds to blood glucose spikes by producing more insulin, a hormone that causes your body to stop burning fat and start burning carbohydrates. It also sends out hunger signals and tells your body to store fat. When you consume lower-GI foods, it helps you to avoid blood glucose spikes, as well as manage your weight and overall health.

Understanding carbohydrates and their effects on your glucose level is important in making good choices. If you are prone to diabetes, have diabetes, are trying to lose weight, or just want to maintain good health then it is a good practice to always select foods with a lower glycemic index. In this postindustrial age, refined foods have become cheaper and more available, thus contributing to the obesity epidemic and increasing the risks of diabetes and heart disease. Food should be consumed wisely and not abused.

What are fats?

Fat is another of the macronutrients and one of the 3 major sources of fuel for our body. It comes from a variety of sources. Most people think of animal fat when this term is used. but many plants are also sources of fat. The section will review how the body uses fat for energy.

Fat, also called adipose tissue, holds your internal organs in place, makes up a large percentage of your brain, and helps to connect your skin to your frame. It is a vital component of the human structure and is only an issue when there is an excessive amount.

The fat you consume is broken down into fatty acids. You may have heard the term "essential fatty acids" (EFAs). These are simply fats that are essential for the body to maintain optimum health. Our bodies cannot manufacture these types of fat, so we must get them in our diets. The two EFAs are called omega-3 (alpha linolenic), which is found in oily fish, and omega-6 (cis linoleic), which is found in vegetable oils. Another fatty acid, called arachidonic acid, is semi-essential. The body can make it provided it has an adequate supply of other nutrients.

EFAs are vital for the health of your heart and circulatory system, brain development and function, as well as many other bodily functions. EFAs are found in safflower, sunflower, corn, sesame, pumpkin, and linseed oils. Other good food sources include green vegetables, tofu, fish (for example, salmon, mackerel, rainbow trout and sardines), and fish oils.

Although all whole, fresh, unprocessed foods contain some EFAs, they must go through many changes as the body breaks them down and refines them into useful substances. We usually take in enough EFAs through the diet but, unfortunately, we also take in other foods that block the breakdown of the EFAs and prevent them from doing their valuable work. These foods include saturated fat, cholesterol, excessive amounts of alcohol, and high levels of sugar.

Fat is either saturated (solid at room temperature) or unsaturated (liquid at room temperature). Most saturated fats are of animal origin (exceptions include palm and coconut oils) and contain high levels of cholesterol, which is another fatty substance present in animal fat. Cholesterol can clog up arteries and restrict blood flow if consumed in excess.

Saturated fat has been associated with heart disease. To restrict your intake of both saturated fat and cholesterol, reduce the amount of meat you eat and always choose lean cuts. Despite popular belief, beef is not exceptionally high in cholesterol and contains a comparable amount as chicken or fish. The total saturated fat content of beef is more than chicken or fish.

After they're ingested, fats are broken down into fatty acids, which are used for development and maintenance of our bodily structure. Certain fats are better than others, but you should always limit your intake to the recommended amounts. An excess of any food source can be deleterious to your health. Stored fat is the body's way of "saving up for a rainy day." In situations where food sources are limited, stored fat can be utilized for energy for up to 40 days. Excessive amounts, however, can limit your life expectancy and lead to the development of chronic diseases.

Micronutrients, Fiber, and Water

Fats, carbohydrates, and proteins fuel our body, but they require micronutrients, fiber, and water to support the body's function. This section will review these nutrients.

Micronutrients are those food components that are needed in small amounts to support the body's functions. They include vitamins, minerals, trace elements, phytochemicals, and antioxidants. They are required in a precise amount: too much or too little can create problems. Most of these must be consumed in our diet. The only exception is Vitamin D, which is made by our bodies though it requires sunlight for production.

There is still much to be learned about the role of the micronutrients. Vitamin and mineral deficiencies and toxicities can be described for many micronutrients, but the effects of insufficient levels are poorly understood. In fact, it is still unclear as to what represents an optimal level for many of these micronutrients. We know that the antioxidant vitamins such as C and E help the body dispose of free radicals (waste product of cellular metabolism), which can damage the cells. However, the role of these micronutrients in cancer prevention and other disease process are only now being intently studied.

Fiber is the component of plant foods that can't be digested. It contains cellulose, lignin, and pectin, which are resistant to the digestive enzymes. Other terms used for it are roughage and bulk. It is an important component of a nutritious diet.

There are two types of fiber: soluble and insoluble. Soluble fiber dissolves in water and helps to regulate blood glucose and cholesterol levels. It is contained in nuts, beans, apples, oatmeal, and other sources. Insoluble fiber does not dissolve. It helps the digestive system to balance water absorption and promotes intestinal motility. This type of fiber is contained in whole grain products, wheat, brown rice, legumes, and many vegetables.

It is recommended that we consume 14 grams of fiber per 1,000 calories. This is approximately 25 grams per day for women and 38 grams per day for a man. Fiber has been proven to lower insulin levels, improve the lipid profile, control glucose levels, and lower blood pressure. Research has demonstrated that a diet high in fiber will decrease heart disease and diabetes.

Water: Most of us take it for granted, but have you ever taken a moment to stop and think just how important water is to you? For the human body, water is truly a vital resource. You can go weeks without food but only 5 to 7 days without water. When the water in your body is reduced by just 1 percent, you become thirsty; at 5 percent muscle strength and endurance decline significantly and you become hot and tired. When the loss reaches 10 percent, delirium and blurred vision occur. A 20 percent reduction in water leads to death.

There is no more important nutrient for our bodies than water. No other substance is as widely involved in the processes and makeup of the body. A man's body is about 60 percent water, and a woman's is approximately 50 percent. The human brain is about 75 percent water.

Every day, we lose 2 to 3 quarts of water through urination, sweating, and breathing. Because many of the processes within the body rely greatly on water, it is important we replace our fluids regularly to compensate for this loss.

When you are planning a nutritious diet for yourself or your family, remember the micronutrients, water, and fiber. You will get most of the micronutrients you need if you eat the recommended amount of fruits and vegetables, but pay attention to special needs during pregnancy, in children, or for the elderly. Make sure you factor in plenty of water and don't forget to include at least 25 grams of fiber.

Diet Basics

Your diet should reflect your health and fitness goals and will constantly change over time. A 50-year-old sedentary man should not eat the same as an adolescent athlete. Your choice of foods and the amount you eat will be based on your current situation. If you are trying to lose weight you will eat fewer calories and those who need to gain weight will eat more calories. If you have an office job and do very little physical activity, you need fewer calories to fuel your body than someone who has a physically demanding job or is a marathon runner. Developing children need more fuel than a mature adult.

Your health status should also drive your food choices. Individuals with hypertension should avoid foods high in sodium while those with diabetes should have a diet that restricts carbohydrates and avoids added sugars. Someone who has heart disease needs to be more conscious of the types of fats in his diet compared to the individual whose cholesterol is 125.

Not everyone can afford to buy expensive cuts of meats or even the tastiest vegetables, however it is worth your while to plan your meals with your budget in mind. Shopping at a farmer's market might be cheaper than trying to buy vegetables from the corner store. Purchasing food items in bulk and storing (or freezing) the excess is a wise investment. There are plenty of ways to make healthy eating affordable.

Not everything we want is available and there is plenty that we can't afford. Planning a diet that is tasty and healthy can be a challenge and of course if we enjoy eating the food then we are more likely to do this in the long run. However, taste isn't a necessity. There are some foods that we just need to eat because it's good for us, even if it isn't good to us. Just try to strike a balance and always veer on the side of nutritious.

There are numerous reasons to start a diet, and many of us have undertaken a diet to achieve any number of goals. The need to diet can be triggered by a number of things: an upcoming event, inability to wear clothing, a new health problem, the search for a new partner, a sports competition, or maybe you have just learned of the importance of a nutritious diet. In either case, the key to success is information.

Many people abuse their bodies through months or even years of poor diets, often without realizing it. They follow the latest fad diet, taken in by false promises and unrealistic expectations. Some of these diets result in drastic weight loss over a short period of time, which seems great but can be dangerous. The other drawback is the temporary nature of the loss. As soon as you finish the diet, you start to regain the weight and often put on even more than before the diet.

Regaining weight is counter-productive and can have a negative effect on your self-esteem and confidence. It usually occurs because you were not on a well-balanced diet, and your body wasn't getting the amount of food it needed to stay healthy while you were on the plan. In addition, some of the diets are difficult to sustain over time and can lead to a rebound effect where you wind up eating even more calories or unhealthy foods.

Fad diets might be appealing but a truly healthy diet is one that can be sustained over time. If you are trying to achieve one or more of the above goals, then do the due diligence. Investigate proper diets and fitness plans to help you achieve your goals. Know that patience is required, and that it is a marathon, not a sprint. Choose a method that will allow you to sustain the changes for a lifetime.

A Review of Common Diets

Most of us have attempted to diet at some point in our lives. For many the goal is weight loss, but special diets are also available to achieve other health related goals. Some people want to gain weight; others want to gain muscle while still others want to maintain a healthy weight. There are diets for health-related problems such as diabetes, hypertension, and heart disease as well as for the environmentally aware individual who wants to lead a healthy life. This section reviews some of the more popular safe and successful diets.

DASH Diet

DASH was developed to provide an option for managing high blood pressure without the use of medications. Its logic is based on the fact that potassium, calcium, protein, and fiber lowers blood pressure. It is nutritiously complete, safe, and useful for those who are trying to prevent or manage diabetes and heart disease. It consists of a daily intake of 4 to 5 fruits, 4 to 5 vegetables, 2 to 3 servings of dairy, and less than 25 percent fat. It is proven to lower both the systolic and diastolic blood pressure.

TLC Diet

Therapeutic Lifestyle Changes, or TLC, is a diet created by the National Institutes of Health. It is designed to promote cardiovascular health by lowering the cholesterol levels through decreasing the amount of saturated fat in the diet. It focuses on encouraging lifestyle changes in both diet and exercise. It requires motivation and serves as a guide for healthy living.

Mayo Clinic Diet

The Mayo Clinic designed this diet to assist in the development of a lifelong healthy eating habit with the objective of weight loss. If followed, it boasts a 6 to 10-pound weight loss in the first 2 weeks. It combines direction with education. It tells you what to do to lose the weight, then provides you with the information necessary to make good food choices.

Mediterranean Diet

This diet has many advantages. It is a diet that is high in fruits, vegetables, nuts, and seeds. Olive oil is its source of monounsaturated fat. Other characteristics include low-to-moderate wine consumption, small amounts of red meat, and low-to-moderate fish, poultry, and dairy intake. Populations with this type of diet have a lower-than-average incidence of cardiovascular death, cancer, Parkinson's disease, and Alzheimer's disease.

Weight Watchers

Weight Watchers is a commercial success because it is smart and effective. Experts praise it because it is nutritiously complete and safe. Other advantages include an emphasis on group support, plenty of fruits and vegetables, and the built-in indulgences that help with the sweet cravings.

Vegetarian Diets

Although this wasn't among the ranked diets it is important to note that vegetarians have a lower incidence of obesity, heart disease, hypertension, and diabetes. The best outcomes are with those lactovegetarians who consume milk and dairy products.

There are numerous resources available to help to make appropriate food choices. Based on your needs and personal goals, you should be able to find a plan that is right for you. Remember the goal of good nutrition is to maintain a healthy body so you can function at the highest level possible.

THE BOTTOM LINE

- Energy and nutritional requirements vary depending on your stage of development and activity levels.
- Carbohydrates, fats, and proteins are the energy nutrients.
- Calories measure the amount of energy our bodies use to function.
- There are numerous reasons to diet and it is important to clearly define your objectives when you decide to diet.

Fitness

The second thing you can do to ensure good health and live a long life is to stay as fit as possible. Fitness is the state of being in good health. To be fit also means the ability to survive and reproduce. There are numerous studies that show the role of regular exercise in preventing chronic illness, increasing life expectancy, and improving the quality of life. This section will focus on the value of physical fitness and how to incorporate it into your life.

<u>Why exercise?</u>

There are many reasons to exercise, and everyone has their own objective when starting a regimen. No matter the reason, just start. Exercise should be a part of daily life, as routine as eating and sleeping. The benefits are many and the reasons reviewed below aren't the only ones.

The main reason most adults start to exercise is to control their weight. This may be driven by an individual recognition of the need to lose weight or on the advice of a physician. Exercise works because it causes your body to burn calories. Weight loss occurs if your body burns more calories per day than it consumes. Regular exercise helps to achieve this by burning calories during physical activity but also by building muscle that in turn burns more calories, even if you are not exercising.

Aesthetics is another reason. Some people don't like the way their bodies look and embark upon a journey to reshape it. Losing fat and gaining muscle can significantly change the appearance of one's body and is easily achieved with the proper exercise regimen.

Another major reason to exercise on a regular basis is to maintain good health and prevent medical problems. Regular exercise has been proven to lower the risk of heart disease and stroke by 35 percent or more. It decreases the risk of type 2 diabetes and colon cancer by 50 percent and even decreases the risk of breast cancer. There is a 30 percent reduction in premature death, depression and dementia in those who exercise regularly. Consistent physical activity also reduces the risk of falls and fractures in the elderly. It is clear there are numerous health benefits to regular exercise.

People who exercise on a regular basis just feel better, sleep better, and have an improved mood and more energy. Exercise is the ideal therapy to help combat stress and manage symptoms of depression. There are even reports that exercise helps those with substance abuse problems stay clean. It may be hard to imagine and the effect isn't immediate, but improved mental health and sense of well-being is one of the benefits of being fit.

The demands of daily life vary from person to person. Some people have physically demanding jobs and need to be fit to make a living. The need to walk long distances, lift heavy objects, or even to remain highly focused are requirements for many jobs. Staying physically fit may be the competitive edge you need to get a job, keep a job, or be promoted. Busy mothers and fathers know the energy it requires to chase a toddler, and stay-at-home spouses can attest to the physical exertion required to run a household. Performing consistent and regular exercise can aid you in meeting the demands of your daily life.

Some people exercise simply because they enjoy it. Golfers, tennis players, hikers, bikers, martial artists, and others do it because it is an enjoyable part of their life. Those who are professional or amateur athletes must be fit in order to compete. An appropriate physical fitness regimen can make the difference between winning and losing and the ability to continue their chosen profession.

Those who participate in regular fitness activities because they enjoy it are more likely to remain physically active over the long term. If you want to start a regular regimen, chose an activity you enjoy and try to find a partner. This will increase your chance of being successful.

What are you trying to do?

Have you decided to start regular exercise? If so, ask yourself why. What are you trying to achieve? The answer to this will help you choose the proper fitness regimen. The recommended route may be different if you want to lose weight, maintain your weight, build muscle, or improve your endurance.

Selecting a regimen targeted toward achieving your objectives increases your chance of being successful. For instance, a person who wants to gain muscle will need to focus on strength training, while someone who wants to lose weight would need to start with an aerobic training routine designed to burn calories. Walking for 45 minutes or more 4 to 5 times per week would meet this objective. It is also important to reassess your regimen periodically as there is value in changing up your fitness routine. Your goals may also change over time, and if this is the case then the regimen would also need to be changed.

There are many resources to help. The Internet, health magazines, and your health care provider are good initial sources. The American Heart Association and the Centers for Disease Control are reliable sources of information about physical activity directed toward improving your health. Local fitness centers and physical fitness experts such as personal trainers can also provide you with direction if you are starting your journey to fitness. If is important to consult your physician before starting a fitness routine if you are older or have medical problems.

Exercise Basics

Different exercises achieve different results. It is important to be familiar with the different types to make the proper choices. The science of exercise can be quite complex and understanding the basics is required to get started.

Aerobic exercise increases the heart and respiratory rate. Examples include walking, running, jumping rope, riding a bike, and other activities that require exertion leading to increased work by the heart and increased breathing effort. This is because muscles need more oxygen to meet the exercise's demands. The more you do this type of exercise, the more efficient the body becomes at using oxygen and other energy sources, and the easier it becomes to perform the same amount of work. The results can be seen when you go from taking 15 minutes to run a mile to running one in 9 minutes or when you appreciate that it becomes easier to perform a specific exercise for a longer period. The results are improved heart health, increased endurance, and the capability of performing better and longer.

Strength or resistance training is designed to build muscular strength. These types of exercises, including weight lifting, resistance training with bands and calisthenics, are all ways to target and stimulate the muscles. There are numerous ways to incorporate muscle strengthening into your exercise regimen. Women are more prone to losing muscle mass as they age. Strength training is one way to prevent this from happening. Strong muscles also protect the bones and prevent fractures, especially in older women who may have the risk of experiencing a fall. Strength training is a crucial aspect of a quality fitness routine.

Flexibility and balance exercises are also important components of regular exercise. Stretching improves the flexibility of the body and protects against injury to muscles, joints, and ligaments. It is important to do this regularly, and especially before and after exertional exercises.

Balance training isn't discussed much and most people are not aware of how bad their balance is until they attempt these types of exercises. Improved balance is especially important as we age as poor balance is the primary cause of falls. The older you get, the more you can appreciate the importance of flexibility in combating stiffness and preventing injury, as well as good balance and improved coordination.

An ideal fitness regimen incorporates elements of aerobic, strength, flexibility, and balance training. All of this is required for a comprehensive physical fitness program that achieves the goal of good health. You can develop a regimen that includes each of the elements 1 to 2 times per week. Many exercise programs achieve all objectives in one sitting. Pilates, martial arts, and certain group exercise programs are examples.

How to Exercise

If you have never exercised before, the best advice is to start slow. You should discuss your plans of starting an exercise regimen with your physician if you have medical problems or are older. If you don't have any risks or health concerns, start something as soon as you can.

Walking is a great way to get started. You can start walking 15 minutes a day (depending on your fitness level), 4 to 5 days per week and then gradually increase the amount of time you walk up to 1 hour. Write down how much you've done and how much you would like to do. Lay out a clear plan. If you do this, then you are more likely to be successful. Once you have achieved your goal then set a new goal. Let's say you have been walking 1 hour per day 4 to 5 days per week for the past 3 months. You might want to consider, running for 2 to 3 minutes and then walking in between. Many people who've never exercised have found that they can go from walking to running 3 to 5 miles or more. It's achievable! Walking is only an example. You may decide to swim or bike or even hike. The principle is the same: Start slow and gradually increase.

What if you have been doing this for several months now and are getting bored or haven't achieved your goals? Then it is time to mix it up. Incorporate some strength and flexibility training. Stretch before and afterwards. Do some pushups. Start with 3 pushups and after a few months you may surprise yourself and find that you can do 25. Sign up for the yoga class or invest in a Pilates video. Many group fitness classes are streamed online. Join a gym. This is a great way to socialize and meet new people. Learn a new skill. If you've always wanted to learn to swim now is the time to do it. Grab a friend and take up tennis. Did you want to do martial arts when you were younger and never had the chance? It's never too late to start. Most cities and towns will have a local gym that offers these types of classes, and martial artists are some of the most gracious and welcoming athletes in the world. They love having beginners!

Whatever you decide to do, set goals. You need to define what you are trying to achieve so you will know when you have, giving you something to look forward to and celebrate when you've accomplished it. Chose something you enjoy doing and try to stay consistent. Life events, work demands or even injury may interrupt your routine, but find a way to get back to it. You may have to reassess your regimen or even change your goals, but this is life. Be open-minded and flexible. Remember the most important thing is to be consistent. Make exercise a routine part of your life.

THE BOTTOM LINE

- Physical fitness should be a part of your daily routine just like eating and drinking.

- The choice of an exercise routine should be based on your fitness goals.
- Regular exercise can extend your life!
- The best way to ensure success with a fitness regimen is to do something you enjoy.

Substance Abuse

The overuse or abuse of certain substances contributes to a significant amount of premature deaths and illnesses. If you smoke or drink alcohol in excess, then stopping this is the third action you can take to increase your chance of living a full and healthy life. Other substance abuse can contribute to health problems, but a coverage of these is beyond the scope of this book. This section will discuss two of the most common: cigarette use and alcohol abuse.

Cigarette Use

Whenever I see a patient who is perfectly healthy but smokes, my advice is always the same, "the best thing you can do for yourself and your family is to quit smoking. The greatest risk to your health right now are those cigarettes." It's true! Smoking can shorten your life by at least 10 years. That's a lot! This section will review the ill-effects of smoking, explain what you are putting in your body when you smoke, review reasons to quit, and describe ways to do it.

Why Smoking Is Bad

What if I told you that the leading cause of death in the U.S. could be prevented in most cases by one simple act? I'm sure you would respond by asking what it is and why people don't do it. Smoking is a bad habit for so many reasons and I believe most people don't understand the full extent of the problems caused by cigarettes.

Smoking cigarettes contributes to 400,000 deaths per year in the U.S. and 6 million worldwide. Fifty percent of smokers will die from a smoking-related illness, and the list of illnesses caused or exacerbated by smoking is quite long. Three of the leading causes of death are related to smoking: heart disease, chronic obstructive pulmonary disease, and many cancers. In fact, 33 percent of the cardiovascular deaths in U.S. are due to smoking. It causes 90 percent of all lung cancers, 80 percent of all chronic obstructive pulmonary disease deaths, and increases the risk of heart disease and stroke twofold to fourfold.

Smoking is associated with cancers of the bladder, lung, cervix, colon, esophagus, larynx, liver, throat, kidney, pancreas, stomach, and others. One-third of cancer deaths are due to smoking. These statistics are astonishing, and have been consistently demonstrated. Smoking is a serious health hazard.

Cigarettes are dangerous during pregnancy, both for the mother and fetus. Cigarette exposure increases risk of preterm delivery, stillbirths, low birth weight, sudden infant death syndrome, ectopic pregnancies, and certain birth defects. It is also known to decrease fertility in men and women. Exposure to smoke is bad in numerous other ways: increasing the risk of upper respiratory problems in children; causing erectile dysfunction in men; leading to premature menopause in women; and contributing to post-operative complications in those who undergo surgery.

There just isn't anything good to be said about cigarettes.

What's in a cigarette?

Cigarettes contains approximately 600 ingredients which, when burned, develop into over 7,000 toxic chemicals. These chemicals are familiar to us all and, if asked, no one would voluntarily consume any of these: acetone, the main ingredient in nail polish remover; acetic acid, like that found in hair dye; ammonia, commonly used in cleaning products; arsenic, which is the active ingredient in rat poison; and methanol, which is used in rocket fuel, are all on that list. But this isn't all. Benzene (in rubber cement), butane (in lighter fluid), cadmium (in battery acid), tar (used to pave roads), nicotine (put in insecticides), formaldehyde (used in embalming fluid), carbon monoxide (car exhaust fumes), naphthalene (placed in moth balls), and lead are all part of the smoking experience. I'm sure you recognize many of these poisons. This is what a smoker or second-hand smoker takes in every time they inhale cigarette smoke.

Effects of Smoking on the Body

Needless to say, cigarette smoke is a pure poison. However, the specific effects they produce help us to understand how all of the diseases described above occur.

Cigarettes are addictive primarily because of the nicotine. It binds to pleasure receptors in the brain to relieve stress and decrease anxiety. It's easy to understand how addiction occurs. Other physiologic effects include increased metabolism and appetite suppression.

Nicotine causes vasoconstriction (narrowing) of the arteries, most notably the coronary arteries, which supply the heart. The results are increased heart rate and increased blood pressure. Nicotine also damages the endothelial cells (cells that line the blood vessels), causes blood to clot more rapidly, and leads to elevated blood cholesterol levels. This state of combined hypercoagulability, dyslipidemia, endothelial dysfunction, and coronary artery vasoconstriction is the blueprint for a heart attack. This same recipe will also produce a stroke.

The lungs have cells with little hair-like projections called cilia that line the airways. These cilia are responsible for trapping and removing harmful substances from the inhaled air, preventing it from reaching the deeper air sacs and the body. The air sacs deep within the lung are where oxygen is passed from the inhaled air into the blood stream. Within the blood, hemoglobin is responsible for transporting the oxygen throughout the body. Cigarettes affect these vital structures. The smoke kills or paralyzes the cilia, destroys the air sacs, inflames the airways, and interferes with oxygen uptake in the blood. The consequence is recurrent respiratory infections, asthma, emphysema, chronic bronchitis, and poor oxygen perfusion to the tissues of the body.

The poisons in cigarettes are also carcinogenic, causing cancer by destroying the genetic material of cells and preventing proper repair. If this genetic material cannot repair itself then rogue cells develop and become cancerous. The damage to tissue extends to the blood system, leading to poor healing and a weak immune system. Muscle and bone have decreased turnover and difficulty developing, leading to increased muscular fatigue and weakness.

From an aesthetic perspective, the consequences are just as dramatic. Smoking decreases skin elasticity and contributes to the development of wrinkles. Aging effects become visible as early as 30 years. There isn't an organ in the body that is free of the effects of cigarette smoke.

It's Never Too Late to Quit

It's possible to quit even if you have smoked for years. Many people have found the motivation to quit, sometimes by learning about the hazards of smoking and sometimes for other compelling reasons. The good news is that the benefits of smoking cessation can be seen even in those who have smoked for years. Once exposure to the poisonous smoke has stopped, the body can heal itself. Hopefully, the following list of reasons to quit will provide you with some inspiration.

The onset of health problems or a health scare can be a wake-up call. Illness is a reminder of our mortality and there's no better motivation than the recognition that your time on Earth may soon be over. For some this realization makes quitting cigarettes easy. The best way to fight a cigarette-induced illness is to stop the exposure.

The prospect of having a family makes many people view life and risk taking differently. Smoking is indeed a risky behavior. The love of a spouse or child is one of the strongest motivations in the world. Most parents would do anything to keep their child safe. Quitting cigarettes is the most important step you can take to ensure a healthy pregnancy. Keeping your children away from second-hand smoke is the next most important step to ensuring their good health as they grow.

A pack of cigarettes costs $5 to $10 per pack, depending on where they are purchased in the U.S. If you smoke one pack per day, then you would spend over $2,000 per year. That's $20,000 over ten years. That's a lot of money.

It's not a hard decision. Smoking is unhealthy, causes premature death, is harmful to your children, and is expensive. If you can't do it for yourself then do it for your family. It's never too late!

How to Quit

There are numerous ways to quit and many resources available to help. The American Lung Association is great place to start and provides comprehensive information on line. Below is an overview of some of the methods.

Cold turkey is probably the most difficult way. This entails just stopping. The success rate is quite low at 4 to 7 percent, and it probably works for those people who are not really nicotine dependent.

Behavioral therapy involves a combination of actions designed to help wean you off the cigarettes and to reinforce habits that facilitate quitting. This may involve counseling, a strategy to decrease the number of cigarettes over time with an identified stop date, and a plan to manage cravings. Identifying triggers that lead you to smoke and creating a plan to manage this is also a part of the strategy. If stress is a trigger, finding other ways to deal with stress would be one action. Some people only smoke when they drink alcohol or go out with certain friends. These are other triggers that can be eliminated.

Nicotine replacement therapy is an effective strategy for quitting smoking that can be purchased without a prescription. These gums, patches, inhalers, lozenges, and sprays help manage the nicotine craving and allow you to be free of cigarettes. The nicotine dependence can then be managed through a weaning process whereby you gradually decrease the amount of these replacement therapies.

Effective medications are available to help you quit. They work on the brain chemistry to counteract the effects of nicotine. Zyban (bupropion) and Chantix (varenicline) are two examples of FDA-approved products available in the U.S. These medications require a prescription so you will need to consult with a physician to start this therapy, but this also allows an opportunity to discuss the pros and cons of the treatment and to consider alternatives for trying to quit.

Some of the therapies above may be used in combination to help you achieve your goal of quitting cigarettes. If you try and fail, don't give up. Try again. The benefit of being smoke-free is worth it. Keep trying!

Alcohol

People worldwide indulge in the pleasure of having a drink. Wine, beer, whiskey, liqueurs, and other forms of alcohol have been enjoyed for centuries, and moderate consumption has some health benefits. Drinking 1 to 2 glasses per day of red wine, for example, appears to decrease the risk of some health problems, like cardiovascular disease. Drinking more than 4 to 5 drinks on any given occasion qualifies as alcohol abuse. This is when the danger occurs.

"Alcohol use disorders" is the term used to describe those who abuse alcohol and those who are alcoholics. The problem is worldwide and affects women, men, and children. Approximately 16 million adults and 679,000 adolescents in the U.S. suffered from this disorder in 2014. Alcohol-related events kill approximately 88,000 people per year in the U.S., which makes it the fourth leading cause of preventable deaths.

Alcohol Abuse

Alcohol abuse occurs when a person's pattern of drinking places them at risk of harm. This harm could be physical, emotional, or financial. Intoxication affects judgement and people under the influence may make poor choices which could lead to injury. The classic example is driving under the influence, which could lead to their death and the deaths of innocent people. Getting into fights or being vulnerable to rape or robbery are other dangers a drunk person might encounter. Alcohol abuse can affect relationships and interfere with obligations such as work and school, the consequences of which could include the loss of a job, failing in school, financial ruin, and the destruction of intimate relationships. The other major risk is the development of alcohol dependency, which carries even more serious and sometimes irreversible consequences.

Alcoholism

Alcoholism is a chronic illness. It occurs when a person becomes dependent on alcohol to function. This dependence is both physical and mental. The National Institute on Alcohol Abuse and Alcoholism describes four keys symptoms that defines alcoholism: cravings, loss of control, tolerance to alcohol, and physical dependence. The urge to drink is overwhelming and is nearly impossible to control, they can't stop, and when they don't drink they suffer from symptoms of withdrawal such as nausea, vomiting, and sweating. The longer an alcohol-dependent person drinks, the more drinks they need to consume to relieve the craving and to become drunk. People who experience these symptoms are alcoholics and need help to break the dependence.

Why It Occurs

Some people are more susceptible to dependence than others. Genetics and environmental influences each play a role in whether someone is likely to become addicted or not. Mental health problems also contribute as many use alcohol to ease the pain of depression, anxiety, and other mental problems.

Alcohol stimulates the release of dopamine in the brain, which is a pleasure hormone. Repeated exposure to alcohol affects multiple neurotransmitter pathways in the brain, altering them in a way that increases the need for more and more alcohol. Alcohol withdrawal leads to the development of undesirable symptoms such as nausea, vomiting, anxiety, tremors, and even seizures. Continued drinking is reinforced because alcohol relieves the withdrawal symptoms.

The Dangers of Alcohol

Acute alcohol intoxication affects judgment. Individuals who are inebriated make poor decisions, making them a danger to themselves and others. Motor vehicle accidents, drownings, physical assault, sexual assault, exposure to sexually transmitted infections, and altercations with law enforcement are examples of the many incidents that may result while under the influence of alcohol.

Alcohol is a toxin and those who binge drink place themselves at risk of acute poisoning. Confusion, stupor, coma, seizures, respiratory depression, and hypothermia can occur and result in death if immediate medical treatment isn't undertaken.

There are also long-term medical consequences that result from chronic alcoholism. Excessive alcohol damages body tissues. Chronic exposure to the mouth, throat, and esophagus can cause cancer. The liver is responsible for removing poisons from the body and in this capacity it is chronically exposed. If liver cells are damaged, it can lead to hepatitis, cirrhosis, and liver failure. Pancreas damage can lead to bouts of pancreatitis and diabetes. Gastrointestinal bleeding can result in hemorrhage. Heart failure, life-threatening arrhythmias, and strokes are also known to occur more commonly with alcohol abuse. Any of these events can result in immediate death. One of the saddest things I have witnessed is watching someone die from liver failure.

How to Quit

This is not easy once a physical dependence has occurred. But it isn't impossible. The key is figuring out why you drink. Explore the reasons behind the behavior. Is it social? Then change your social circle. Is it because of an underlying depression? Seek the help of a mental health provider. Those who binge drink may be able to stop simply by making a conscious decision.

If you are at university you can start with the student health center or with your primary care provider. You can talk to your parents or a trusted adult such as a teacher or principal if you are underage. Those who have a physical dependence will need to undertake treatment with healthcare providers that specialize in substance dependence. Resources can be found at local hospitals, the National Council on

Alcoholism and Drug Dependence, the National Institute on Alcohol Abuse and Alcoholism, and the Centers for Disease Control.

THE BOTTOM LINE

- Cigarette and alcohol abuse is a serious health risk.
- Stopping the use of these substances is the most important step you can take to ensure good health.
- It is never too late to quit.

Chapter 9

Cancer: It Can Be Prevented or Beaten!

For physicians and patients alike, the most dreaded word in medicine is 'cancer.' In the past, speaking these words were equivalent to a death sentence. But unlike the punishment of the electric chair or lethal injections, death from cancer can be long, painful and emotionally devastating for the affected person and their loved ones. This isn't necessarily the case today. Many cancers can be prevented and those that aren't can be beaten. This chapter will review the most common cancers in women and outline ways to ensure you don't become a victim.

Breast Cancer

Gigi has always gone to the doctor for her routine visits. This was a habit but she had never inquired as to what tests were done or why. She recently read an article which talked about cancer prevention in women. "Doctor, I just turned 40 and recently learned that I should have some tests to check for female cancers. Would you please explain this to me?" She asks in a lovely Italian accent.

Breast Cancer Prevention

Breast cancer is the most common malignancy in women.[1] Approximately 1 out of every 8 women will develop breast cancer in her lifetime.[2] Certain women are at higher risk than others. What are the factors that place some women at increased risk? Is there anything that can be done to prevent breast cancer? Risk factors for breast cancer are both genetic and environmental. The environmental factors can be modified, thereby potentially reducing the likelihood of developing cancer. Even though there aren't ways to modify genetic risk, there are ways to identify these risks. Treatment options are available to reduce the probability in high-risk groups.

The risk of breast cancer increases with age. Women between 25 to 34 years of age have a 2 percent risk while those 35 to 44 years have a 9 percent risk and those 45-54 have a risk of 20 percent. It increases to 30 percent in women between ages 55 to 64 and is over 43 percent in the groups above this.[2] Combining age with other factors allows for a risk assessment. There are several models available to calculate an individual's risk. The assessment can be done for a 5-year period or the life time risk can be determined.

One of the most commonly used risk assessment tools is called the Gail Model.[3] It combines information on age, age at menarche (first period), age of first live birth, number of first-degree relatives with breast cancer, race, the number of previous breast biopsies, and other factors to determine a woman's risk. Once this is determined an individualized screening and prevention plan can be developed. The screening may entail more frequent mammograms or ultrasounds but could also employ more complex imaging modalities such as magnetic resonance imaging. Of course, in women at higher risk, there is a much lower threshold for evaluating abnormalities.

Modifiable risk factors are those that are not genetic and can potentially be changed. Obesity is one factor. Women with a body mass index greater than 30 are at higher risk. The use of exogenous estrogen, specifically the use of hormone replacement therapy for more than 5 years, leads to an increased likelihood. Women who breast feed are at lower risk. In addition, those who exercise regularly and who consume higher amounts of fruits and vegetables are at lower risk. As with other medical conditions, smoking and excessive alcohol use can increase the risk of developing cancer.

So, even though you can't change your genes, there are actions you can take to prevent breast cancer. These actions can have multiple benefits, including decreasing your chance of developing other life-threatening medical problems. If you are obese or overweight, get serious about reducing your weight. If you are at a healthy weight, focus on preventing weight gain, which occurs easily with aging. Regular exercise and consuming fresh fruits and vegetables are components of a weight loss program so you will be combating risks on 3 fronts. Breast feeding for more than 6 months is beneficial to you in many ways and has lifelong benefits for your baby. Moderating your alcohol intake and quitting smoking are some of the smartest health decision you could make. Finally, if you don't need hormone replacement therapy then don't accept it, and if you do, try to wean off as soon as possible.

Breast Cancer Screening

The goal of breast cancer screening is to detect breast cancer as early as possible. The earlier it is detected, the greater the likelihood of preventing death. Another benefit of screening is that it can also detect other changes that indicate a higher risk of developing cancer in the future. Women who are at greater risk can then be monitored more closely based on their risk assessment.

Breast cancer screening consists of self-breast examination, clinical examination by a physician, and routine imaging, usually with mammography. This section will focus on the recommendations for women at average risk.

There is much discussion as to the benefit of self-breast examination. In general, most physicians suggest that women start examining their breasts in their early 20s. The idea is that you become familiar with your breast and, if there are any changes, you are more likely to notice them earlier. The examination should be done once a month, approximately 1 week after the period. It consists of observation of the breast and palpation (firm pressure) around the entire breast and into the axilla (armpit). The idea is to note any skin or architectural changes and to feel for small lumps. The American College of Obstetricians and Gynecologists recommends a yearly gynecologic examination for all women. The breast examination is a part of this evaluation and essentially consists of the provider observing and palpating the breast.

The institution of routine screening mammography has been the main contributor to the decreased mortality from breast cancer. A mammogram can detect lesions as small as 1 mm in diameter. A lesion this size would not be felt on breast examination and would potentially continue to grow several years before it could be detected by physical examination.

The "sojourn time" is the timeframe from when a tumor can be detected by mammogram until it can be detected by clinical examination. The major factor in this detection time is age, but other factors may play a role. For instance, in women age 40 to 49 years it is 2 to 2.4 years and it increases after this. The sojourn time is considered when making recommendations for routine mammogram screening intervals. The goal is to detect the cancer as early as possible to maximize the chance of a cure.

There are many other factors to consider when recommending screening intervals. The cost of screening and exposure risk are two examples. It is these considerations and perspectives that explain why recommendations may vary among organizations. In the age group 40 to 49 years, over 746 women would have to be screened to prevent 1 death, while in the 50 to 59 group only 351 would need to be screened.[4]

The different organizations concerned with this issue include the American College of Obstetricians and Gynecologists, the American Cancer Society, the National Cancer Institute, and the U.S. Preventive Services Task Force. They recommend screening mammography starting at 40-45 with a recommended interval of 1 to 2 years for this group. After age 75, the decision for routine screening should be based on an individual's life expectancy and health status.

As you can see, the recommendations for routine mammography screening are done from a population perspective and take a number of factors into consideration. Women who are at higher risk of developing breast cancer should consult with a specialist to develop an appropriate screening interval. You should work with your doctor to develop a plan that is rational and feasible.

<u>Medications to Prevent Breast Cancer</u>

All women and some men are at risk of developing breast cancer. There isn't a single factor that guarantees the development of breast cancer, but some are stronger than others. In addition, the factors can have a cumulative effect. There are medications available to prevent breast cancer, but these should only be prescribed for women with specific factors. The side effects and potential for other problems prohibits the use of these medications in women at average or slightly higher than average risk.

Women who should consider using these endocrine therapies are those who fall into the high-risk categories:

- Women with known genetic mutations that lead to breast cancer and who have not undergone a prophylactic

(preventative) mastectomy (the most commonly recognized mutations are BRCA1 and BRCA2)
- Women who have been diagnosed with early contained cancer of the ducts and breast lobes (ductal carcinoma in situ -DCIS or lobular carcinoma in situ-LCIS)
- Women with atypical hyperplasia (abnormal excessive growth) especially over the age of 35
- Women ages 35 to 59 who have a calculated 5-year breast cancer risk of 1.66 percent should be counseled on this option for prevention
- All women over the age of 60 should be considered

Selective estrogen receptor modulators were the first to be widely used to reduce the chance of developing breast cancer. The most commonly used are tamoxifen and raloxifene. They work by blocking estrogen receptors in the breast, preventing the proliferative effect of estrogen on the tissue. In other tissues, they may act as receptor activators, simulating estrogen and thereby producing estrogen-like effects. The other type of medication is aromatase inhibitors, which are relatively new and act by decreasing the circulating levels of estrogen in postmenopausal women.

Tamoxifen is the most commonly used medication to prevent primary and recurrent breast cancer. It decreases the risk of developing cancer by 50 percent. It has anti-estrogen effects in breast tissue but agonistic (triggering) effects in the uterus and other tissues, meaning that women who take this medication have a higher risk of developing endometrial cancer and should be monitored appropriately. Those women also have an increased risk of venous thromboembolism such as a deep vein thrombosis (deep blood clots), pulmonary embolism (blockage in the lungs), and stroke.

Raloxifene was initially approved for the prevention of osteoporosis because of its agonist effects on the bone helping to maintain density.

Like tamoxifen it has an antagonist effect on the breast and is nearly as effective as tamoxifen in reducing the incidence of cancer. The major bothersome side effects are hot flashes and leg cramps. There is also an increased risk of venous thromboembolism.

The aromatase inhibitors include letrozole, anastrazole and exemestane. They block an enzyme whose function is to make estrogens. This therapy is effective in postmenopausal women, lowering the circulating levels of estrogen. In women who are still menstruating there is an opposite effect, and therefore this is not recommended for breast cancer treatment or prevention. The side effects are therefore the typical low-estrogen ones, such as hot flashes, vaginal dryness, joint pain and low bone density. The risk of venous thromboembolism and endometrial cancer is not increased.

Continued research has provided revolutionary therapies for the treatment of breast cancer, improving the survival rate dramatically over the past decade. This is excellent news for the 12 percent of women who will develop breast cancer. Prevention, however, is still the ideal, as no one should have to go through the anxiety, pain, and fear associated with a breast cancer diagnosis. You should see your gynecologist regularly and know your family history. Your doctor can help you assess your risk of breast cancer and direct you to the appropriate provider so you can get the care you deserve.

Understanding BRCA

Breast cancer is the most common cancer in women, and a family history of breast cancer is therefore not unusual. There are hereditary syndromes in which a genetic predisposition increases the likelihood of developing breast and other cancers. This section will focus on BRCA hereditary breast and ovarian cancer (HBOC) syndromes.

BRCA 1 and 2 stand for breast cancer susceptibility genes type 1 and 2. A mutation in these genes makes the affected individual more susceptible to developing breast or ovarian cancer over the course of their life. In women with these mutations, the risk of developing breast cancer by age 70 is 45 to 65 percent and ovarian cancer is 11 to 39 percent.[8] The gene is transmitted in an autosomal dominant fashion, meaning that the child of an affected person has a 50 percent chance of having this gene.

These genes are responsible for most hereditary breast and ovarian cancer syndromes (HBOC). There are other hereditary cancer syndromes that are due to mutations in other genes. However, it is important to understand that inherited genetic mutations are responsible for less than 10 percent of breast and <15 percent of ovarian cancers.

You should be concerned about a possible hereditary genetic mutation if there is a family history of many women (and even men) with breast cancer, especially first-degree relatives. You should be equally concerned if there is a family history of ovarian cancer as well as colon, endometrial, pancreatic, and prostate cancers. The likelihood of a hereditary genetic mutation is also increased if the cancers are diagnosed in younger women.

If you are concerned about the possibility of a familial predisposition to any cancer, you should discuss these concerns with your physician. Genetic testing is available to identify the presence of certain mutations. This should only be done after in-depth counseling as there are many consequences to discovering that you are a carrier.

In women who carry these genetic mutations, many options are available to manage the risks. Breast and ovarian cancer surveillance can be undertaken. Risk reduction surgeries are available. Medication options for chemoprevention have been used as well. The decision to utilize one method over the other is dependent on several factors that should be discussed with an experienced health care provider.

Every woman should have a clinical breast examination by a physician periodically. Breast screening options also include the initiation of mammography at an earlier age and more frequently. Breast imaging can include alternating magnetic resonance imaging with mammography to increase the likelihood of early detection. A combination of pelvic imaging and testing for blood cancer markers at regular intervals are options for ovarian cancer surveillance. These techniques should start at least 5 to 10 years earlier than the age of the youngest affected relatives, or by age 25 for breast cancer surveillance and age 35 for the ovarian cancer surveillance.

Risk reduction surgeries can be done as well. Prophylactic bilateral total mastectomy decreases the risk of breast cancer by 90 percent. Removal of the ovaries and tubes by age 35 to 40 significantly reduces the risk of both ovarian and breast cancer.[9]

Chemoprevention is also an option. Tamoxifen, raloxifene, and aromatase inhibitors are options to decrease the risk of breast cancer. Oral contraceptive (birth control) pills are thought to reduce the risk of ovarian cancer by 50 percent.[10]

A strong family history of breast, ovarian, and other cancers is a sign of a possible hereditary genetic mutation. It is important to recognize this and seek consultation to understand your personal risk. Even though this is a scary thought, remember knowledge is power. If you have this mutation, there are options for decreasing the chance of developing cancer. In addition, this information is vital to the health of other family members, including your children.

THE BOTTOM LINE

- The best treatment for cancer is prevention.
- The next best treatment for cancer is early detection.
- Regular mammograms are the best tool available to detect breast cancer at a stage where it can be easily treated.

Cervical Cancer

Maryam recently arrived to the U.S. and, despite having given birth to 5 children, had never had a pap test. She had become friendly with her new neighbor who had invited her to participate in a cancer awareness event for women. Maryam learned a lot participating in this community event and had come to see me on the recommendation of another friend. "Please tell me what screening test I need to do." She was very clear about what she wanted. I gave her a big smile and sat down to review her medical history. I was so impressed with this woman who had moved from the Middle East, quickly integrated into her community and was eager to take the steps needed to ensure continued good health.

Cervical Cancer Prevention

Cervical cancer is a malignancy of the cervix that is known to often result from sexual exposure to a virus called Human Papilloma Virus (HPV). Once the cells of the cervix are infected it is possible for the body to fight the infection, but this doesn't occur in all women. In some cases, the cervix may undergo precancerous changes and eventually develop cancer. This process can take years, providing an opportunity for early detection of changes and cancer prevention.

Cervical cancer is the third most common cancer in women worldwide and the second most common cancer in women ages 15 to 45.[11] Cervical cancer is caused almost exclusively by HPV infection; its presence has been found in 97 to 100 percent of cervical cancer cases. Women who develop cervical cancer are known to have specific factors. Over 60 percent of them have never received a pap smear or have been inadequately screened. Those who develop cervical cancer have persistent infection with the high-risk HPV types, are heavy smokers, or are immunosuppressed. Cervical cancer screening when done correctly is effective.

Thirty-five of the over 100 HPV types are known to infect the genital tract. The types are categorized as being high risk due to their strong association with cervical and other genital cancers. HPV types 16, 18, 45, and 31 cause 65 percent of the cases of high-grade precancerous lesions. Types 16 and 18 have been implicated in 70 to 80 percent of the cases of cervical cancer and 10 other types with the rest of cervical cancers. Types 6 and 11 are generally associated with low-grade lesions but cause 80 to 90 percent of the cases of genital warts.[12]

Over 20 million adults in the U.S. are infected with the Human Papilloma Virus. It is estimated that the acquisition rate for sexually active adults is 6.2 million per year. Seventy-five to 80 percent of all sexually active adults will become infected at some point in their life. Women, especially younger women, are more likely to be infected, and it is estimated that 60 percent of them will become infected within 3 years of becoming sexually active.

Most HPV infections resolve spontaneously, the majority within 8 months, but some may take up to 30 months. Of women with high-risk HPV types, 15 to 30 percent will develop high-grade lesions within 4 years and the rate of progression to invasive cancer is 1.44 percent during a 2-year period.

Precancerous changes are described as dysplasia and are categorized as low- or high-grade lesions. The low-grade lesions are typically due to an acute HPV infection and usually regress. The high-grade lesions are associated with persistent HPV infection and thus are at greater risk of developing into cancer. This progression can take from 3 to 12 years and occurs in more than 30 percent of the severe dysplasia cases.

Cervical cancer is one of the most preventable cancers. The availability of screening cytology (Pap smear), ability of early detection and treatment of precancerous changes, and recent vaccination means that no woman (especially in developed countries) should die from this cancer. The possibility of eradication of this cancer is within our grasp. Every woman and girl should be given the opportunity to take advantage of screening tests and preventative methods. If detected early, even invasive cervical cancer can be successfully treated.

The addition of HPV testing has made identification of true cervical abnormalities much easier. The known association of HPV virus types with dysplasia and cervical cancer allows for more aggressive management of those at greater risk. If the Pap test has atypical squamous cells and HPV testing reveals the presence of the high-risk virus types, a colposcopy is required. This is a procedure where the tissue of the cervix is examined under magnification. A colposcopy is also required if the Pap reflects any degree of dysplasia.

The early diagnosis and appropriate treatment of cervical dysplasia has been an effective strategy in cervical cancer prevention. When cervical cancer is diagnosed, it is usually in someone who has not had a Pap test in many years. The identification of HPV virus as the causative agent of cervical cancer has allowed the development of a vaccine that has the potential to decrease the incidence of cervical cancer almost entirely as well as decrease the incidence of dysplasia.

Screening

The institution of routine Pap tests has reduced the incidence of cervical cancer by 50 percent over the past 3 decades, but it remains a problem. It has been estimated that there are over 500,000 new cases worldwide each year. There are over 12,000 new cases of cervical cancer and over 4,000 deaths attributed to this malignancy in the U.S. yearly.

Recent understanding of the role of HPV in the development of cervical cancer has led to the development of new screening tools. Even though there are approximately 35 types of HPV that infect the genitals, only some of these are known to cause cervical cancer. Types 16 and 18 are responsible for over 75 percent of the cervical cancers and another 10 types are responsible for the rest. These are described as the high-risk types, and their presence can be determined using a simple swab. Screening for their presence can also be done at the same time as the Pap smear.

The Pap smear collects a sample of cells from the cervix that are examined to identify any potential abnormalities. It is important to remember that the Pap is a screening test. Screening tests tend to over-call abnormalities with the goal of not missing any true abnormalities. The consequence is that there will be many reported abnormal Pap smears that, upon further testing, yield normal cervical findings. On the other hand, the Pap smear is unlikely to miss cervical abnormalities.

The cells taken during the Pap smear are examined for changes that reflect cervical dysplasia or cervical cancer. The reported abnormalities may include atypical squamous cells, low-grade squamous intraepithelial lesions, high-grade squamous intraepithelial lesions (which includes moderate and severe dysplasia), atypical glandular cells, and carcinoma. Further evaluation is dependent on the report. The presence or absence of high-risk HPV types can also influence the decision for further evaluation.

Cervical cancer is one of the few cancers that can be prevented. This is due to the availability of an effective screening program. The combination of screening cytology and HPV testing allows for the prompt identification of high-risk individuals. Once precancerous lesions are identified, effective and low risk treatments can be performed. If detected early, even invasive cervical cancer can be successfully treated. The goal is early detection through screening so that treatment can be provided as early as possible.

Human Papilloma Virus

The Human Papilloma Virus (HPV) is a double-stranded DNA virus that infects only humans. There are over 100 types, and subsets show a preference for incorporating into either cutaneous tissue or the mucosa of the oral or genital regions. The consequences for genital infection are varied, depending on the genotype and the individual's ability to fight off the infection.

HPV is transmitted by skin-to-skin and genital-to-genital contact. Cutaneous warts, skin cancer, anogenital warts, cervical cancer, anal cancer, genital cancers and oropharyngeal warts, and cancer can result. The infection is quite common, but the severest consequences are less frequent. It is estimated that 75 to 80 percent of sexually active adults will acquire an HPV infection of the genital tract. This infection resolves in most and by age 30 the prevalence of the infection has dropped dramatically. It is only the small percentage with persistent infection that is at risk of the most serious consequence, cancer.

There are over 35 specific types of HPV that specifically infect the genital tract. These are divided into low-risk and high-risk types. The high-risk types are associated with the development of severe dysplasia (CIN 2-3) and cervical cancer. The types are: 16, 18, 31, 33, 35, 39, 45, 51, 52, 58, 59 and 68. The low-risk types are not associated with the development of cervical cancer but can cause other problems. Genital warts, also referred to as *condylomata acuminata*, and precancerous changes in the vulva, anus, and birth canal result from these infections.[13]

HPV types 16 and 18 are responsible for over 75 percent of the cervical cancers. HPV types 6 and 11 cause over 90 percent of the genital warts. Abnormal Pap smears due to HPV infection and genital warts are a major cause for gynecologic office visits as well as emotional distress. Although less common, cancer of the anus and oropharynx can also result from these infections. HPV infection can place a significant burden on the affected individual, potentially even causing death if unrecognized and untreated.

The knowledge that HPV causes cervical, genital, and oropharngyeal cancers has paved the way for more effective screening and prevention. The Pap smear and appropriate management of abnormalities has led to a significant reduction in cervical cancer incidence over the past 3 to 4 decades. The development of the HPV vaccine has now provided us with a new first-line weapon in the fight against cervical and other cancers.

Human Papilloma Virus Vaccination

There are 3 HPV vaccinations currently available: a quadrivalent type named Gardasil, a bivalent type called Cervirax, and the newest one on the market, the nine-valent vaccine called Gardasil-9. The quadrivalent vaccine is designed to protect against infection from HPV types 6, 11, 16, and 18, while the bivalent vaccine protects against types 16 and 18. The quadrivalent vaccine was designed to prevent infection from the viruses that contribute to most precancerous cervical lesions as well as to genital warts. The bivalent vaccine focuses on cervical cancer prevention only. The nine-valent vaccine provides immunity against HPV types 6, 11, 16, 18, 31, 33,

45, 52, and 58. This new generation of vaccine provides coverage for more of the HPV types that cause urogenital cancers.

The vaccinations have proven to be 97 to 100 percent effective in preventing cervical cancer. The quadrivalent vaccine has also been shown to prevent 99 to 100 percent of genital warts and other precancerous lesions of the female genital tract. The nine-valent vaccine provides the same level of protection. These vaccines are recommended for girls starting at age 11 or 12, and the quadrivalent vaccine is recommended for boys of the same age. The vaccine can be started as early as age 9, and should be offered as a catch-up for all candidates through age 26. There are some potential benefits for women who fall outside this range and studies are currently underway to address other groups.

The vaccine is typically given in a series, like other vaccinations. After the initial injection, the second vaccine should be administered after 2 months, and the last 6 months after the first vaccine. The side effects are the same as other vaccines and include both local and systemic symptoms. The local symptoms occur between 1 and 5 days post injection and include pain, swelling, erythema (reddening), itching, and a hematoma (black and blue mark) at the injection site. The systemic symptoms can occur 1 to 15 days post-injection, and include headache, fever, body aches, nausea, and dizziness. Headaches were reported in approximately 20 percent of recipients and the other symptoms occurred in less than 10 percent.

Does the vaccine provide life-long protection or does it need to be repeated in the future? This is a commonly asked question, and the vaccine trials were designed to answer it. Immune memory describes the body's reaction when it sees an infectious agent to which it has previously been exposed. Typically, the immune system's response is rapid and strong. It produces a high level of antibodies to fight this recognized foe. The HPV vaccine studies showed that after 5 years the level of detectable antibodies was quite low, but if the body is shown a portion of the HPV virus the reaction is immediate. The level of antibodies produced was even higher than the initial response seen after completing the vaccination series.

Vaccinations have been widely used for over a century, and even longer for select infections. They are an effective means of primary prevention, and the HPV vaccine has been proven to work in the same fashion. This is the strongest weapon available in the battle to prevent cervical cancer, and it has the potential to even eradicate this cancer. All women and girls should take advantage of this preventative method.

THE BOTTOM LINE

- Early detection and treatment can prevent cervical cancer. Regular Pap test is recommended for the early detection of cervical cancer.
- HPV, or Human Papilloma Virus, causes the vast majority of cervical cancers. A large percentage of women are infected with this virus but only a small percentage will develop cancer.
- HPV vaccination is available to prevent infection of certain types of Human Papilloma Viruses.

Colorectal Cancer

"Doc, I want to thank you." These were the words Queena used to greet me as I walked into the room. She was here for her postoperative examination. "You're welcome," I said, "but there isn't a reason to thank me for doing my job." I gave her a warm smile and asked how she had been doing. "My colorectal surgeon said that I owe you my life, so you deserve special thanks." She said this with tears of gratitude in her eyes

Queena had been referred to see me for severe anemia. Her primary care physician had done an exam and found a pelvic mass. He diagnosed her with uterine fibroids and thought this might be causing heavy periods and thus anemia. On our first visit, I performed a complete history and learned she did not have heavy bleeding with her menses and a pelvic ultrasound revealed that she had a large pedunculated fibroid with an otherwise normal size uterus. I did a rectal examination and a hemoccult test, which showed there was blood in her stool. I referred her to a colorectal surgeon who performed a colonoscopy and found a large mass in her colon that was an early stage cancer. After counseling, Queena elected to undergo the recommended bowel resection and I removed the pedunculated fibroid. Now she was doing great and didn't need any additional treatment, only a colonoscopy every 3 to 5 years.

Understanding Colorectal Cancer

Colon cancer is a malignancy of the large intestine, or colon, and rectal cancer occurs in the rectum, which is the straight portion of the distal colon that leads to the anus that regulates defecation.

The term "colorectal" refers to both areas. Colorectal cancer is the second most common cause of cancer deaths in the U.S. and the second most commonly diagnosed cancer in women worldwide. This is a potentially beatable cancer because of the knowledge of its development and the availability of effective screening tests.

The digestive system consists of many parts. The digestive process starts in the mouth and stomach, where enzymes break down food into smaller particles. The small intestines are then responsible for the absorption of the nutrients. This is a complex process that involves the exchange of electrolytes and fluid.

Once the absorption of nutrients has taken place in the small intestine the remaining substance passes into the colon. This material goes through the cecum to the ascending colon then to the transverse colon and down through the descending colon into the sigmoid. From the sigmoid it travels into the rectum where it will wait until it can be evacuated through the anus. This passage allows for the final absorption of electrolytes and water before the waste product is expelled from the body. Cancer can occur at any of these points.

Most colorectal cancers arise from adenomas. Most of these adenomas are polyps, but not all. Approximately two-thirds of polyps are adenomatous with the potential to develop cancer, while the other third are hyperplastic and don't develop into a malignancy. The adenomatous polyps typically grow from small to large and then transition to dysplasia, a precancerous state. The transition from dysplasia to cancer can take at least 10 years, thus providing a large window of opportunity to remove the precancerous lesions.

Preventative care medicine recommends screening in those at risk, such as people over the age of 50 and those with a family history of colorectal cancer. The screening is designed to detect signs of an early cancer allowing for early treatment and removal of precancerous lesions before they have an opportunity to develop into cancer.

<u>Who gets colorectal cancer?</u>

Colorectal cancer is the third most common cancer in women and ranks third in causes of cancer death in women in the U.S. It is a common cause of cancer death in all sexes around the world.

The death rates have decreased over the past 20 years but there is still an opportunity to decrease the death rates further.

The incidence and death rates of this cancer vary throughout the world. Many factors influence this, such as life expectancy, diet, nutritional status, and screening. In the U.S., incidence has dropped each year over the past 2 decades due to improved screening and early diagnosis, but the death rate is still quite high. Once diagnosed the chance of dying from this malignancy is about 33 percent.[2] This high death rate is primarily because many people do not undergo routine screening. More than 50 percent of those diagnosed have not undergone any of the recommended screening tests. This means that the cancer is advanced at the time of diagnosis.

The lifetime incidence of colorectal cancer is approximately 5 percent, and more than 90 percent of these cancers occur after the age of 50. It is unusual for a person to have this cancer before the age of 40. After the age of 40 the risk of developing it is about 1.5 percent. The risk increases to 3 percent after 50 years of age and over 5 percent after 60.[2] Other risk factors for colorectal cancer include poor diet, lack of exercise, obesity, and smoking. The risk is also higher in people who don't undergo colorectal screening. Other notable risk factors include genetic predisposition, family history, and race. In the U.S., African Americans are at higher risk of developing this cancer.

Most cases occur sporadically rather than in individuals with an inherited susceptibility, though there are known hereditary colorectal cancer syndromes. Familial adenomatous polyposis and hereditary non-polyposis syndromes are the most commonly recognized and account for about 5 percent of the colorectal cancer cases. These syndromes also increase the risk to the individual of developing other cancers such as endometrial, ovarian, and stomach. In the absence of a genetic mutation, a family history of this cancer in a first-degree relative will increase the risk by twofold. Other risk factors include prior abdominal radiation and a personal history of inflammatory bowel disease (Crohn's and Ulcerative Colitis).

There are known protective factors. People who exercise regularly, use aspirin or non-steroidal anti-inflammatory medication, and eat certain foods are less likely to develop colorectal cancer. Diets high in fruits, vegetables, fiber, and calcium but low in red meat, animal fat, and cholesterol appear to protect against colorectal cancer.

Beating Colorectal Cancer

Over the past couple of decades, an increased understanding of development and treatment has led to improved prevention, early diagnosis, and survival. The tools are available to prevent even more deaths from this devastating disease.

The symptoms of colorectal cancer are not specific, but may include bloating, abdominal pain, and blood in the stool. Sometimes the symptoms are so severe that hospitalization is required. An advanced cancer can cause intestinal obstruction, hemorrhage, peritonitis, and even sepsis. Investigations may uncover a cancer as the cause, but it may be too advanced to cure.

Screening tests are available and designed to detect early signs of a malignancy long before it causes any notable problems. There are a few screening tests available, and the recommended options will be dependent on factors such as availability, cost or coverage, provider or patient preference, and risk factors. Most people should start screening at age 50, but those at higher risk should start earlier. Testing the stool for occult blood is a simple way of discovering the presence of microscopic blood, which might indicate an early cancer. If this is found, you would require further testing.

A sigmoidoscopy is an endoscopic procedure to visualize the descending colon, sigmoid, and rectum, but it does not evaluate the transverse and ascending colon. Imaging tests such as a barium enema have also been used, but those only allow visualization of the last portion of the colon. The gold standard is the colonoscopy, which visualizes the entire colon and allows for the removal of any polyps that may be found. This test is both diagnostic and therapeutic in the sense that it can remove growths, thus preventing the development of cancer.

The recommendations for those at average risk are fecal occult blood tests yearly over the age of 40, a sigmoidoscopy or barium enema every 5 years, or a colonoscopy every 10 years if the results are negative. For those with a family history, a genetic predisposition, known adenomatous polyps, and other specific risks, the screening intervals will be more frequent. The ideal test is the colonoscopy, but the potential risks and benefits as well as the cost should be weighed when selecting a screening test.

Colorectal cancer can be beat. It is important to understand your personal risks and seek the advice of your healthcare adviser. Taking advantage of the available medical screening test is truly a matter of life and death.

Other Gynecologic Cancers

Vivian, a very healthy 67-year-old, comes to see me for a routine gynecologic exam and ask, "Which cancer will I get doc?" I respond, "That's an unusual question, what makes you think you will get a cancer?" She explained to me that at her age she knew something medical was bound to happen and since her blood pressure and cholesterol were normal and she didn't have diabetes then it must be cancer.

Understanding Endometrial Cancer

Endometrial Cancer is a malignancy of the lining of the uterus. The term uterine cancer is also used, but this also includes malignancies that arise in other areas of the uterus. It is the fourth most common cancer in women and the most commonly diagnosed cancer of the female genital tract in developed countries. In developing countries, it is second only to cervical cancer. It has a 95 percent 5-year survival rate when detected early and given prompt treatment.

The annual risk of developing endometrial cancer is approximately 8 percent for women over the age of 50.[2] Most endometrial cancers develop because of excessive exposure to estrogen. There are many external and internal factors, which contribute to this increased exposure.

The high survival rate is primarily due to its early presentation. Abnormal uterine bleeding is the first sign of endometrial cancer and typically occurs in 75 to 90 percent of all cases. An abnormal cytology on a Pap smear or an incidental finding after a hysterectomy are others ways it is detected

Abnormal uterine bleeding has many presentations and can have numerous causes. Bleeding in a postmenopausal woman is most certainly abnormal and should be evaluated immediately. Other signs of abnormalities include prolonged periods, excessive bleeding, irregular or intermenstrual bleeding, and bleeding after intercourse. Evaluation under these circumstances is strongly recommended.

Other problems can cause abnormal bleeding, thus the assessment should include testing to evaluate all probable causes. A complete history and physical examination, a pregnancy test in reproductive-age women, complete blood count, and pelvic imaging are the most commonly used tests. An endometrial sampling is the definitive way to determine if a malignancy is present. This can either be by pipelle sampling done in the office or a dilatation and curettage done under anesthesia in an operating room.

In postmenopausal women, an ultrasound to measure the thickness of the endometrial lining can be very helpful in determining the need for sampling. This is a useful tool because an office sampling may not be feasible due to the changes that occur in the reproductive tract after menopause.

Women who develop abnormal uterine bleeding should seek the care of a gynecologist promptly, as should women who are postmenopausal and have any bleeding. Even though the idea is frightening, an early diagnosis is the key to survival in women with endometrial cancer.

Causes of Endometrial Cancer

Endometrial cancer results from malignant changes in a variety of different cell types within the uterus. Thus, endometrial cancer is not a single entity and therefore is likely to have a number of potential causes. There is still much more to be learned about this cancer, even though great strides have been made. It is the most commonly diagnosed cancer of the female reproductive system and the one with the best prognosis as it typically is discovered early in its course.

Endometrial cancers can be grouped into 2 types. Approximately 80 to 85 percent are described as Type 1. They have endometriod histology and are described as grade 1 or 2. This means that they are not aggressive cancers. They usually result from excessive estrogen exposure and typically show precancerous changes before developing to a malignancy. The cancers are quite responsive to treatment and the chance of cure is quite high.

Type 2 endometrial cancers include serous, clear cell, mucinous, squamous, transitional cell, and undifferentiated types, as well as grade 3 endometrioid. They are aggressive cancers that spread rapidly and therefore have a poor prognosis. These tumors are often high grade with an unclear cause, but do not appear to be related to estrogen exposure, and often there isn't any evidence of a precursor lesion, which would lend itself to early diagnosis.

Much of what is known about the epidemiology of endometrial cancer refers to the Type 1 cancers. Many factors contribute to their development. These include exposure to chemicals or radiation and genetic predisposition, but excessive estrogen exposure is the hallmark of Type 1 cancers.

Estrogen stimulates the lining of the uterus to grow, preparing for implantation of fertilized egg. If pregnancy does not occur, a cascade of events is triggered which leads to a drop in estrogen levels and then a withdrawal bleed, which is menstruation. If a woman is not ovulating monthly, the lining of the uterus will continue to grow as estrogen levels remain high. This continuous growth may result in abnormal changes, which could lead to the development of endometrial cancer.

Endometrial tissue that is exposed to continuous excessive estrogen undergoes a gradual transition from normal to abnormal. During this transition, the tissue has a typical appearance that allows the identification of precancerous changes. These precursor lesions are described as hyperplasia. The gradual transition has been described by grading the hyperplasia. Simple hyperplasia is the lowest level and complex is the highest. If there is evidence of atypical cell components, it can be described as atypia. The presence of complex hyperplasia with atypia is the final step before cancer. If this is found on biopsy, there is a high chance that cancer may also be present. Surgical removal of the uterus can prevent the development of endometrial cancer if hyperplasia is discovered.

Most endometrial cancers are easily treated because they have an identifiable precursor lesion and cause classic symptoms that should lead to early diagnosis. It is therefore important to recognize these symptoms and see your gynecologist as soon as possible for a thorough evaluation.

Risk Factors for Endometrial Cancer

Risk factors are certain elements that seem to be associated with a problem. These associated factors help identify causes. As with most cancers, age tends to be the most notable risk factor. The risk of endometrial cancer increases with age and is more common in postmenopausal women.

The other major risk factor is estrogen. This factor appears to be causative in more than 80 percent of the cases of endometrial malignancy. Thus, any condition that leads to an excessive amount of estrogen can contribute to the development of endometrial cancer. Such conditions include obesity, chronic anovulation, exogenous unopposed estrogen use, and medications that have estrogen-like effects on the endometrium.

Obese women have a greater amount of circulating estrogen due to the peripheral conversion of precursor chemicals to estrogen by adipose (fat) cells. This estrogen can stimulate disproportionate endometrial growth, which could then lead to abnormal cell changes and cancer. In addition, the excessive estrogen has a negative feedback on the central reproductive regulator center in the brain, suppressing ovulation and preventing the normal cycle of progestin production, which normally has a protective effect on the endometrium and drives menstruation. Without menstruation, the tissue continues to grow and has an opportunity to undergo malignant changes.

Women who take estrogen replacement therapy without the use of progestin to counter its effect on the endometrium are more likely to develop cancer. This is described as "unopposed" estrogen. Women who elect to take hormone replacement therapy should make sure they also receive progestin in addition to the estrogen if they still have their uterus. Finally, tamoxifen, which is used to treat breast cancer, has an estrogen-like effect on the endometrium and is capable to causing endometrial cancer. As previously mentioned, abnormal bleeding is the first sign of an endometrial malignancy.

Anovulation, infrequent menstruation, can lead to the development of endometrial cancer via the mechanism described above for obese women. If ovulation does not occur, the normal cycle of menstruation is prevented, allowing continued unopposed growth of the endometrium.

The other factors that have been found to be associated with the development of endometrial cancer include: having never been pregnant, early onset of menstruation, and late menopause. There are also hereditary cancer syndromes that increase the risk of cancer. The most commonly identified is Lynch Syndrome, which is manifested as hereditary nonpolyposis colorectal cancer and confers a lifetime risk of endometrial cancer of 27 to 71 percent. It also increases the risk of ovarian cancer.[17]

Protective factors are those that decrease the risk of developing a disease. Protective factors for endometrial cancer include pregnancy, oral contraceptive pills, and a later age of child bearing.

Opportunities for prevention also include weight control and promptly seeking care if you have irregular menstrual cycles.

Endometrial cancer is one of the more common gynecologic cancers. As with all medical problems, awareness, early detection, and prompt treatment are the keys to saving lives.

Beating Endometrial Cancer

Endometrial cancer, like many other medical conditions, can be beat. But you can't defeat an enemy if you don't know you have one and if you are not properly armed to fight the battles. Awareness of the problem is the first step. The second step is action. When you realize you are a potential target for this malignancy then you should seek help.

An early diagnosis is one key to beating endometrial cancer. The most common first symptom is abnormal bleeding in reproductive-age women and any unexplained bleeding in a postmenopausal woman. If you experience either of these, you should see your gynecologist as soon as possible to investigate the cause. Most of the time the symptoms are due to other causes and not cancer, but it is important to be seen. Most cases of endometrial cancer are caught early: 68 percent are usually Stage 1-2, 20 percent are typically Stage 3, and only 8 percent are stage 4, which involves distant metastasis. If caught during the early stages, a simple hysterectomy may be the only treatment needed. If caught at later stages, the chance of survival is significantly lower.[2]

Early treatment of problems like abnormal bleeding, irregular cycles, and hyperplasia can prevent the development of cancer. Skipping cycles can also lead to the development of hyperplasia and subsequent endometrial cancer. This does not apply to the occasional skipped menstruation, but rather in cases where the irregular cycles have gone on for years and not been addressed. If you have a diagnosis of hyperplasia, it is important to follow the treatment regimen and follow-up instructions provided by your doctor. Finally, if you have prolonged menstruation, bleeding in between your menstruation, or any abnormal bleeding it is important to see a gynecologist as soon as possible.

Endometrial cancer, hyperplasia, irregular cycles, skipped periods, and abnormal bleeding can potentially be prevented. If you are overweight or obese, losing weight can be helpful. Excessive body fat contributes to estrogen excess and the subsequent development of hyperplasia and, potentially, cancer. If you have irregular cycles or skipped periods, see your gynecologist to develop a plan to regulate your cycles. If you are not happy with the treatment, don't just stop it; schedule a follow up visit to discuss other options.

Endometrial cancer is the fourth most common cancer in women and the most commonly diagnosed cancer of the female genital tract in developed countries. It is also one that can be easily treated. There aren't many cancers that can be cured or even prevented, but many of the gynecologic cancers can be beaten. Awareness, early detection, and prompt treatment are the keys to beating endometrial cancer.

Precancerous Lesions of the Genital Tract

The cancers of the vulva and vagina typically develop over a long period. Normal cells undergo a transition to cancer, and this transitional stage is described as pre-cancerous. This represents an opportunity to prevent the development of cancer. The precancerous lesions in the vulva are described as vulvar intraepithelial neoplasia (VIN) and in the vagina it is described as VAIN.

The acronym VIN is used to describe high-grade lesions, classified as VIN usual type and VIN differentiated type. The usual type includes the warty and basaloid types as well as those that have features of both and is associated with HPV, while the differentiated type is not associated with HPV. The term "unclassified" is used to describe the lesions that don't fit into either category.

The VAIN category represents pre-cancerous changes or squamous cell atypia of the vagina. VAIN 1 is present when the lower third of the cells are affected, VAIN 2 when two-thirds of the thickness is involved, and VAIN 3 is when more than two-thirds of the tissue thickness has atypical cells. VAIN 3 is also described as "carcinoma in-situ," and the next stage would be invasive cancer. VAIN is much less common than VIN or CIN (cervical intraeptithelial neoplasia).

The risk factors for VIN usual type and VAIN are the same. They include infection with HPV, smoking, and immunosuppression. HPV types 16, 18 and 31 are the oncogenic types associated with the high-grade lesions, while types 6 and 11 are associated with the lesions previously classified as VIN 1. The risk factors for differentiated VIN are the same as those for HPV negative vulvar cancer and tend to be older age and a history of vulvar dystrophies.

The precancerous lesions associated with HPV infection tend to be multifocal and multicentric. If these lesions are found in one site then there is a good chance that they are present in other areas of the female genital tract. Sixty percent of women with VIN or VAIN will also have CIN while 10 percent of women with CIN 3 will have VIN or VAIN.

Once a diagnosis of VIN and VAIN is made, immediate treatment should be given to prevent cancer from developing. This diagnosis also suggests an increased risk for similar lesions in the cervix, so a screening Pap and/or HPV testing is recommended. Early detection is the key to prevent cancer of the female genital tract.

Diagnosis of VIN and VAIN

Cancers of the vulva and vagina represents about 8 percent of female genital tract malignancies. They typically present as pre-cancerous lesions, which provide a window of opportunity to prevent the transition to cancer. Not all pre-cancerous lesions develop into cancer, but their presence should prompt further evaluation and treatment due to the increased lifetime risk of genital tract cancers.

Symptoms of vulvar pre-cancerous lesions (VIN) are like the symptoms of vulvar cancer, including itching, burning, pain with urination, visible lesion, palpable nodularity, or perineal pain. The symptoms of pre-cancerous lesions of the vagina (VAIN) are also like those for vaginal cancer. Some women do not have any symptoms at all and the lesion is found at the time of a routine gynecologic examination. Other symptoms include postcoital bleeding, abnormal bleeding, and an unusual discharge.

The presence of any of these symptoms should prompt immediate evaluation by a health care provider. The precancerous lesions can have a variable appearance. They can be raised or flat, and the color can be white, red, pink, brown or grey. Any abnormal lesion should be biopsied. If there is any suggestion of a precancerous lesion, then a complete evaluation of the genital tract is strongly recommended, including a Pap smear. The presence of these lesions suggests that other lesions might be present either in the same area or in other places along the genital tract.

Not all precancerous lesions will progress to cancer. The availability of information on VAIN is limited but the evidence suggests that less than a third will progress over time while more than two-thirds will regress. If left untreated, 9 percent of VIN cases will progress to cancer. Even if treatment occurs approximately one-third will recur over time and 4 to 8 percent of these will develop to invasive cancer. This cancer can occur at the site of treatment, but could also be at a distinctly separate site.[20]

Even though the diagnosis of a pre-cancerous lesion doesn't mean you will develop cancer, urgent attention is required and long-term care is needed to prevent an unwanted outcome. Risk factors for the development of cancer and for recurrence include immunosuppression, smoking, and persistent HPV infection. Those who are at higher risk require more frequent surveillance. Effective treatment is available to prevent the development of cancer and now there is a vaccine, which can minimize the risk of HPV infection.

Management of VIN and VAIN

Pre-cancerous lesions of the vulva and vagina are a sign of oncogenic (tumor-causing) activity within this tissue. A large percentage of such lesions will resolve spontaneously, but it is impossible to know which ones may progress. The goal of treatment is to prevent the development of invasive cancer. The risk of cancer is not limited to the current site of the change but includes other areas of the genital tract, extending into the distant future. VIN and VAIN require long-term care and surveillance.

The choice of treatment is dependent on many factors. The location and size of the lesion must be considered when choosing therapy. Treatment of a single lesion is different than treating multiple lesions at different locations. Finally, individual factors should be considered. The treatment of a first lesion might be different than a recurrent lesion. A healthy person might be treated differently than someone who is immunosuppressed. These and other factors are usually considered when a provider makes recommendations for treatment.

Simple excision of the involved area is the most common and logical treatment choice. This allows for complete removal and confirmation of the diagnosis. The depth of involvement can be described, which may be grade 1, 2 or 3, and the worst case could include a detection of an early invasive cancer. This is more challenging when the lesion is high in the birth canal or covers a large area. In such cases, a more radical excision may be required. Laser ablation is often used when there is a wide area of involvement.

Treatment with medications is also an option. Aldara (imiquimod) cream is a popular treatment because it is easy to use. It can be self-applied and has minimal side effects. It is described as an immune response modifier with antiviral and antitumor effects. Other options for treatment include 5-fluoruracil and radiation treatment.

Prevention is always better. The greatest risk factors for the development of these cancers are smoking and Human Papilloma Virus (HPV) infection. If you smoke, quitting is the best thing you can do for yourself. If you are a candidate, consider receiving the quadrivalent HPV vaccine, which is highly effective in preventing cancer of the female genital tract resulting from HPV infection.

Understanding Vulvar Cancer

Vulvar cancer is the fourth most common cancer of the female genital tract. It develops when the epithelium of the genital area undergoes neoplastic changes (abnormal growth) that persist over time. This is called pre-cancerous or intraepithelial lesion. When it starts to invade into deeper structures then it is described as invasive cancer. Even though this cancer is less common, it can be equally devastating as the consequences of both treatment and no treatment are potentially life altering.

Vulvar cancer accounts for 5 percent of genital tract malignancies and tends to occur in older women, with the average age of diagnosis being 65. This is probably due to the slow-growing nature of this malignancy. The pre-cancerous phase can last for years, with some lesions regressing over time. Only a small percentage of precancerous lesions develop into cancer. The risk factors for the development of vulvar cancer include postmenopausal status, smoking, immunosuppression, HPV infection, and certain vulvar dystrophies.

Even though vulvar cancer is less frequent than the other genital tract cancers, awareness is still important. The initial symptoms can be vague or even absent. Treatment can be simple and straightforward if it is detected early. Prevention is even better. The steps are simple:

Avoid or stop smoking, get the HPV vaccine if you are at risk, and see your gynecologist on a regular basis for a routine check.

Vulvar Cancer Types

The vulvar tissue is composed of many cell types and cancer can arise from any of them, producing different types of malignancies at the site. Most of the tissue is made up of squamous cells, and squamous cell carcinoma accounts for 90 percent of the malignancies of the vulva. Typically, when the term vulvar cancer is used, it is referring to these squamous cell carcinomas.

Other cells that make up the vulva include columnar cells, which are typically found in the glands of the genital tract, cells from the basement membrane of the skin, melanin-producing cells (melanocytes), and cells that produce the tissue support structures. The common types of cancer from these cells include melanoma, sarcoma, basal cell carcinoma, adenocarcinoma, and Bartholin's gland carcinoma. These types are not as common and will not be discussed in this section.

There are two types of squamous cell malignancies in the vulvar area, distinguishable by their cause, or "etiology." The simplex type–keratinizing and differentiated—typically is found in older women and often occurs in the setting of chronic inflammation that occurs with conditions like vulvar dystrophies. The classic type is warty, or "Bowenoid," and associated with HPV infection. It is found in younger women and is easily diagnosed in an earlier stage due to its appearance. HPV types 16, 18, and 33 are most often associated with this type of vulvar malignancy. One variant, called verrucous carcinoma, has a cauliflower-like appearance. It is slow-growing and rarely metastasizes but causes local destruction of adjacent tissue.

Of course, the issue with all cancer is its potential to spread, interfering with normal organ function. Vulvar cancer spreads by local extension to adjacent structures, distorting their appearance and interfering with their function. The cancer cells can also spread through the lymph system, passing through the lymph nodes or via the blood stream.

Vulvar Cancer Treatment

The vulva area consists of the labia majora, labia minora, clitoris, mons, introitus, vestibule, and urethra meatus. Its function is to direct the urine stream, protect the genital tract, and serve as a sensory organ for sexual arousal. A cancer in this area can directly affect all these functions and spread to adjacent and distant structures.

Once a cancer diagnosis is made the next step is to determine the extent of its spread. This process is called clinical staging and helps determine both the treatment options and the prognosis. This consists of a complete history and physical examination, including a pelvic examination, taking note of abnormal lesions and even enlarged lymph nodes. A more detailed evaluation of the genital tract may include a colposcopy and vulvoscopy to examine for spread or other foci of cancer in the cervix and rest of genital tract. A cystoscopy provides a detailed urethra and bladder evaluation, while an anoscopy allows for visualization of the anus. Additional imaging may be advised depending on the examination findings.

The final staging is confirmed by surgical evaluation. A biopsy can describe the depth of the lesion. Additional surgery, which may be both diagnostic and therapeutic, includes removal of the vulvar structures and a lymph node biopsy. The extent of these procedures is determined by the location, size, and evidence of spread. A stage IB cancer is greater than 2 cm in diameter. Stage II cancers have spread to the vagina, urethra, or anus. Stage III has spread regionally beyond these structures, and Stage IV is distal spread outside of the pelvic region. Metastasis is found in approximately 5 percent of cases at initial diagnosis.

Surgical treatment is possible in those cases that are diagnosed early. Radiation and chemotherapy are additional treatments that may be utilized if the cancer is at an advanced stage. An early diagnosis allows for easier treatment, and the likelihood of success is much higher. You should consult a gynecologist if you have unusual genital symptoms or a lesion. In some cases, it may require persistence on your part to find the answer, but don't be afraid to be an advocate for your health.

<u>Vaginal Cancer</u>

Malignancy of the vagina is extremely rare, representing 3 percent of cancers of the female genital tract. This is probably the least-discussed reproductive organ cancer, yet it too can be devastating, causing significant morbidity and mortality.

The incidence of vaginal cancer is about 1 per 100,000 women. There are approximately 4000 new cases per year in the U.S. and 900 deaths. It is unusual for cancers to occur here as a primary site. Most of these are metastases from other sites, such as the cervix, endometrium, vulva, ovary, breast, or other organs.[1]

The mean age of women who develop vaginal cancer is 60. Older women are at a higher risk of developing this malignancy, but other risk factors include smoking and multiple lifetime sexual partners. As with genital tract cancers, human papilloma virus (HPV) appears to contribute to a significant number of these cancers. HPV antibodies have been identified in more than 50 percent of women with this malignancy. Thus, women with a history of severe cervical dysplasia,

HPV infection, and vulvar cancer are also at higher risk of developing vaginal cancer[22].

The symptoms of this cancer vary but include postmenopausal bleeding and post-coital bleeding. Other complaints include a watery, blood-tinged, or malodorous (bad-smelling) discharge. A vaginal mass maybe noted by the woman or she might report symptoms of the urinary or gastrointestinal tract. These symptoms may include pain with urination or defecation, blood in the urine or stool, and frequent urination or constipation. Pelvic pain maybe described occasionally and this is usually means the cancer has spread beyond the vagina.

Some women will not have symptoms and the cancer might be found on routine gynecologic examination. The examiner may unexpectedly find a mass, plaque, or an ulcer. The masses can be nodular or fleshy, and may grow beneath or above the surface. Any suspicious lesion should be biopsied and a thorough assessment of the entire genital tract should be performed because these cancers can be multifocal and multi-centric.

There is also a tendency for these cancers to occur at specific sites in the vagina. Fifty percent occur on the posterior wall, as opposed to the anterior wall, while 50 percent occur in the upper canal, 20 percent occur in the mid-canal, and 30 percent occur in the lower portion. The importance of a routine gynecologic examination cannot be overstressed. Many early cancers of the female genital tract are detected on routine screening. Every woman, even those past the reproductive age should have a gynecologic exam on a regular basis.

Management of Vaginal Cancers

A vaginal malignancy can be difficult to detect. Even though it is uncommon, it contributes to significant morbidity and mortality.

The symptoms can be non-specific but any abnormal bleeding, unusual discharge, or genital masses warrant further evaluation by an experienced clinician.

The majority of cancers of the vagina derive from squamous cells. They are usually associated with HPV infection and tend to be slow-growing. There is a small chance that a malignancy is present in other sites within the vagina or in other areas of the genital tract. Other types of cancers of the vagina include sarcoma, melanoma, and adenocarcinoma.

Adenocarcinoma represents the major type of vaginal cancer in young women, and the major factor for this is in-utero exposure to diethylstilbestrol (DES). Adenocarcinoma can develop at the site of adenosis, endometriosis, periurethral glands, or other embryonic elements but the anterior wall of the vagina is the usual site.

The appearance of an early cancer of the vagina can be a nodule, ulcer, or a mass. A biopsy of the area of concern can confirm the diagnosis. Once this is done, a thorough evaluation is required to see if the cancer has spread and how far. This is called staging. The staging is based on a physical examination, pelvic examination, cystoscopy, proctoscopy, imaging, and lymph node biopsy.

Most vaginal cancers are discovered in their early stages: 36 percent in Stage I and 22 percent in Stage II. Stage III is present 11 percent of the time and Stage IV 14 percent[22]. Treatment is determined based on the stage. Stage I is usually treated with surgery, which includes resection of upper vagina, radical hysterectomy, and lymph node dissection. Intracavitary radiation therapy is also an option for this stage. Stage II is usually treated with chemotherapy followed by radical surgery. The treatment of advanced stage cancers is determined by a number of factors and is beyond the scope of this book.

Survival rates for Stage I is about 84 percent, Stage II is 75 percent, Stage III and Stage IV is around 57 percent. The best chance for survival is with an early diagnosis.[22]

Vaginal cancers can be difficult to detect early due to their location. Women should have routine gynecologic examinations, which include an inspection of this area. Any abnormal bleeding, discharge, or growth should prompt an immediate visit to a health care provider. In most cases, the cause will be easily managed and is usually due to a benign process but being proactive and seeking early care could make the difference between life and death.

<u>Understanding Ovarian Cancer</u>

Ovarian cancer is a malignancy of the female reproductive organ, the ovaries. This diagnosis typically strikes fear in all affected due to the poor prognosis. However, not all ovarian cancers are the same, and the best way to fight this disease (and others) is to understand the problem.

Ovarian cancer arises from the various cell types that make up the ovary. This complex organ has a multitude of functions and therefore has many different cells designed to carry out these functions. The ovaries produce eggs for reproduction and therefore harbor the genetic material that is responsible for creating life. The cells surrounding the germ cells also produce a variety of hormones that play a vital role in supporting a pregnancy.

Ovarian cancers tend to fall into two types: epithelial or germ cell cancers. Within these types are a variety of subtypes. Epithelial cancers represent 90 percent of cases of ovarian cancer. The most common types are serous, mucinous, endometrioid, and clear cell types. The germ cell cancers and other uncommon types represent 10 percent of the ovarian cancer. The prognoses for these vary and depend on the type, specific cellular characteristics and the stage at the time of diagnosis.

Ovarian cancer is the leading cause of death from a gynecologic malignancy. Per the Centers for Disease Control, 22,000 ovarian cancer cases occur every year and it is estimated that more than 14,000 women will die from it.[24] This is a death rate of about 63 percent.

Even though the risk is low, the high death rate makes it a disease of great concern. The 5-year survival of ovarian cancer is about 60 percent, and this is primarily due to late diagnosis. Unfortunately, the survival rates have not improved significantly over the past 30 years, despite advances in other areas of cancer treatment.[2]

More than 75 percent of the cases are diagnosed at an advanced stage and this contributes to the poor prognosis. Unlike breast and cervical cancer, there isn't a screening test available that will allow for early detection. Unlike endometrial cancer, there isn't an early sign that helps doctors to detect this cancer early. The symptoms of ovarian cancer can be vague to none. The slow-growing cancer can be present for years without being detected, and by the time symptoms are present it is usually too late.

The likelihood of developing ovarian cancer is low. Some individuals have factors that place them at higher risk than the average women. It is important to see your gynecologist on a regular basis for routine gynecologic examinations, and, of course, if you have unusual pain or discomfort that is persistent.

Beating Ovarian Cancer

Is it possible to prevent ovarian cancer? Is it possible to successfully treat ovarian cancer? The answer is yes, but it isn't easy. This is the most common cause of death of all gynecologic malignancies even though the lifetime risk is less than 2 percent. This is because ovarian cancer is difficult to detect early. When ovarian cancer is found at Stage I, the 5-year survival rate is 92 percent. When it is found at Stage II is 73 percent, and at Stage III and IV the 5-year survival drops to less than 30 percent.

Ovarian cancer is a silent killer. There are no early warning symptoms and there isn't an appropriate screening test available. In most cases the presenting symptoms are vague and described as pelvic discomfort, pain, fullness, or bloating. These symptoms can be due to a number of causes and are usually not taken seriously. Many studies have been done to see if certain blood and imaging test can effectively detect early cancer. Unfortunately, these tools are not beneficial on a large-scale basis like the mammogram and Pap smear have been.

There are 3 major factors that increase a woman's chance of developing ovarian cancer: age, family history, and the presence of a genetic predisposition. Ovarian cancer tends to occur in women ages 50 to 59. Women in this age group should be more concerned about the vague symptoms mentioned above and doctors who care for these women should have a low threshold to evaluate these symptoms more aggressively.

A woman's chance of developing ovarian cancer increases threefold when there is a first- or second-degree relative with ovarian cancer. This risk is even higher with multiple family members with this malignancy or even breast, endometrial, and colon cancer. There are several familial genetic syndromes that increase the risk of ovarian cancer and, in some cases, this lifetime risk can be as high as 25 to 50 percent. Genetic testing is available, and women should be concerned if they have multiple family members with these cancers or relatives diagnosed with the cancers before age 50.[8]

The risk of ovarian cancer has been found to be lower in certain women. Women who have had pregnancies, breastfed, underwent a tubal ligation or hysterectomy, and took oral contraceptive pills have a lower risk. Birth control pills have been shown to decrease the lifetime risk of ovarian cancer by 50 percent in women who carry certain genetic mutations.[25]

Women who have a genetic predisposition or who are at higher risk, have a number of options. They can have a specifically tailored screen with a combination of blood tests and pelvic ultrasounds every 6 to 12 months to detect early changes. They can strongly consider having their ovaries removed between the ages of 35 and 40 or once they have completed their childbearing. In addition, they can elect to take oral contraceptive pills to reduce their risk. Women who are over the age of 50 should consider having their ovaries removed if given this option when undergoing surgery for other indications.

Ovarian cancer is typically found at an advanced stage where treatment is difficult. It is possible, however, to target certain high risk groups to minimize their chances, and there are a number of other actions that decreases the risk of women in general. The key to beating ovarian cancer is early detection and prevention and this is possible for many.

THE BOTTOM LINE

- The older you get, the greater your chance of developing cancer.
- Ovarian cancer is the one gynecologic cancer that is difficult to diagnose in the early stages.
- The urogenital cancers are less common and typically present with an abnormal lesion or bleeding.
- You should see your gynecologist if you have any urogenital bleeding that is not related to menstruation.

Chapter 10

Pelvic Floor Problems

Some of the least-discussed and more devastating consequences of childbirth are pelvic floor problems. This chapter will provide an overview of the more common ones. Detailed discussion of some of the less common problems is beyond the scope of this book.

Jenna stops me in the hallway as I am seeing my post-surgical patients. She is a quality manager at the hospital and was performing quality rounds. "Dr. Howard, exactly what is a pelvic floor?" I am taken aback by this question so I ask, "What makes you ask about the pelvic floor?" She explains that she had started to experience some pressure in her genital area and had gone to see her primary care physician who told her that her pelvic floor was weak and to do some kegel exercises.

What is the pelvic floor?

The pelvic floor refers to the structures at the bottom of the pelvis that work together to maintain the anatomical position of the pelvic organs while allowing those organs to perform their functions. These structures include the pelvic floor muscles, the vagina, the rectum, the urethra and the connective tissue that hold these organs together.

The pelvic floor muscles are called the "levator ani" muscles (individually the coccygeus muscles). This group of muscles extends from the pubic bone anteriorly to the sacrum, posteriorly and laterally from the right to the left pelvic bones. It forms a shelf of support that is penetrated by the urethra, vagina, and rectum.

The levator ani muscle maintains a constant tone that keeps the vagina closed and maintains support for the urethra and rectum. This muscle relaxes during urination and defecation to aid in the elimination of urine and stool. The levator ani can contract involuntarily to inhibit an undesired bladder contraction or to delay defecation. This muscle can also be contracted voluntarily to achieve the same goals.

The pelvic nerves direct the function of the pelvic floor, allowing the structures to work in coordination. The bladder remains relaxed to allow urine sent from the kidneys to fill and expand it. The urethra, on the other hand, is kept contracted to allow storage of urine without leaking. When nerves in the bladder signal to the brain that it is time to urinate, the individual can take their time and make a trip to the toilet. Once she is ready, the brain can then send a signal via the nerves that it is ok to empty. The bladder then contracts and the urethra and pelvic floor relax allowing elimination of urine. If the person isn't ready to urinate but the bladder insists, then the pelvic muscle can contract telling the bladder to quiet down until a more appropriate time. A similar communication process occurs when the rectum is full and communicates that it is time to defecate.

If these nerves are damaged, pelvic floor problems may result. The muscle itself can also be damaged leading to pelvic floor dysfunction. Childbirth is the primary cause of pelvic floor damage. The stretching of the vagina during delivery can stretch the nerves and tear the connective tissue and muscles. Healing and repair take place, but long-term damage may be the consequence for some. Pelvic surgery and accidents that damage the pelvis may also contribute to the development of pelvic floor problems.

All muscles deteriorate with time and disuse. We don't routinely exercise or voluntarily use the pelvic floor muscles. Muscle damage from childbirth can be compounded by time, and disuse leads to the gradual development of pelvic floor dysfunction with age.

Pelvic Floor Disorders

Pelvic floor disorders are the result of childbirth or insults to the pelvic floor, such as injury or surgery. They include bladder and rectal problems as well as disorders of support. The nerves that supply the pelvic floor direct the function of the bladder and rectum. The connective tissue holds the organs in place. The bladder, uterus, vagina and rectum are all in close proximity and share nerves and connective tissue. Damage to these nerves and connective tissue can affect these structures.

Prolapse, the shifting out of place of an organ, results when there is a problem of pelvic support. Both the uterus and/or the vagina can prolapse, though the degree of prolapse can vary from mild to severe. In the most severe cases of vaginal prolapse, the vagina can bulge through the vaginal opening and be as large as a grapefruit. If the anterior vaginal wall prolapses, the bladder can follow. This is described as a cystocele. If the posterior vaginal wall prolapses, the rectum will bulge forward and sometimes out the vaginal opening. This is called a rectocele. The apex of the vagina can also prolapse in women who have had a hysterectomy. This is referred to as vaginal vault prolapse. Treatment is typically surgical.

Bladder disorders include urinary incontinence, urinary frequency, urgency, and incomplete voiding. Leaking urine can result if the urethra is malfunctioning or if the bladder is contracting when it's not supposed to. This leakage may require pad use and, for some, multiple changes of pad per day. Constantly needing to urinate or experiencing severe urgency of urination can be quite disruptive and may affect quality of life. Less common is the inability to empty the bladder completely, leading to urinary tract infections, which can lead to kidney infections if untreated. Treatments for this group of problems include medication, physical therapy, and surgery in the most severe cases.

Problems with defecation can be due to a rectocele or may also be due to problems with the rectum. If the anal sphincter is damaged at childbirth, fecal incontinence might result. Nerve damage can lead to emptying problems and incontinence as well.

Pelvic floor problems are complex. Many women experience these problems. Evaluation by a skilled health care provider is recommended so that appropriate treatment options are made available.

Prevention of Pelvic Floor Problems

The best approach to pelvic floor problems is prevention. But what can be done to prevent pelvic floor disorders?

There are a few things that can be done during pregnancy, after pregnancy, and for the rest of our lives that may prevent or minimize pelvic floor disorders.

- Pelvic floor muscle exercises or 'kegels' can be done during pregnancy and immediately postpartum to prevent urinary incontinence. Exercising the muscles in the postpartum aids in muscle recovery and prevent atrophy later in life.
- Perineal massage during the third trimester can facilitate stretching of the perineum (posterior vagina), thereby

decreasing the risk of severe lacerations such as those that tear through the anal sphincter.
- Avoid constipation to prevent straining and stretching the pelvic floor.
- Avoid activities that place undue stress on the pelvic floor, such as extreme heavy lifting.

Health care providers can work with pregnant woman to potentially prevent pelvic floor problems. They can:

- Avoid episiotomy if possible. Episiotomy is the greatest risk factor for third- and fourth-degree lacerations (tears through the anal sphincter and into the rectum).
- Avoid instrument deliveries, such as with forceps, which also increase the risk of severe laceration.

Consider a cesarean section for women who are at high risk of developing urinary incontinence or if a difficult delivery is suspected. Some women already have urinary incontinence prior to pregnancy. These women are at high risk of postpartum incontinence.

What can be done if you already suffer? If you are in the early stages then some of the preventative measures mentioned above—regular pelvic floor muscle exercises, avoiding constipation, avoiding heavy lifting—may also help minimize progression of these problems.

You should discuss any concerns about the health of your pelvic floor with your obstetrician, especially if you are concerned about the potential impact of vaginal delivery.

Urinary Incontinence

"Dr. Denise, I feel like a baby! I'm wetting myself all the time and need to wear a diaper when I exercise. I need your help!" Sarah exclaims. She was 45 years

old, had delivered four children vaginally, and had just started exercising to lose the 30 pounds she had gained over the past 10 years.

Urinary Incontinence

Urinary incontinence is a condition in which there is an involuntary loss of urine. This may occur with a stressful event such as coughing or laughing, or it may occur when one develops the urge to urinate and leaks urine prior to making it to the bathroom. In some cases, a woman may appreciate that she is wetting herself but is not able to identify the inciting factor. There are different types of urinary incontinence. This section will focus on the 3 types that are more prevalent in otherwise healthy women.

Stress urinary incontinence occurs when there is leakage of urine because of a sudden increase in abdominal pressure. Coughing, laughing, sneezing, jumping, exercising, walking, or sudden movement can all cause this kind of sudden increase. Urge incontinence occurs when there is urine leakage associated with a sudden strong urge to urinate. When this occurs, the urge to urinate cannot be suppressed and urine is forced out before reaching the toilet. In many cases, a woman may experience both types of incontinence. The term "mixed incontinence" is used to describe this problem.

Urinary incontinence occurs in close to 50 percent of women.[1-3] The prevalence is higher in older women and in women who have delivered their children vaginally. The many shelves of protective pads and undergarments seen in the grocery stores, supercenters, and pharmacies are a testimony to the extent of this problem.

Major risk factors for this condition are childbirth, pelvic trauma, and obesity. This problem can be exacerbated by muscle disuse, certain medical conditions, aging, and weight gain. The decision to seek care is usually dependent on the severity of the problem as well as its impact on one's quality of life. A sedentary woman may have infrequent episodes of stress urinary incontinence but a woman who exercises may have many more occurrences. This woman can either elect to stop exercising or seek care. A woman who stays at home most of the time can empty her bladder frequently, thereby avoiding episodes of urinary urgency. On the other hand, a woman who is socially active and always on the go may not have the opportunity to urinate more frequently thus she is more likely to experience episodes of urge incontinence. She can elect to curb her social life or seek care.

A comprehensive evaluation is required to identify the problem and to make recommendations for treatment. Urogynecologists, or "Female Pelvic Medicine Specialists," are clinicians trained to care for women with pelvic floor disorders such as urinary incontinence. The specialty is now referred to as Female Pelvic Medicine and Reconstructive Surgery. Certain gynecologists and urologists also have an interest in caring for women with urinary incontinence. It is important to identify a specialist who cares for a large volume of women with these problems so that you can be provided with a thorough evaluation and offered a full range of treatment options.

Stress Urinary Incontinence

How does it occur?

Stress urinary incontinence affects up to 30 percent of adult women.[1-3] The severity can range from leakage of a few drops of urine once or twice a month up to leakage of larger amounts several times a day. Occasional leakage of a few drops can be annoying, but recurrent, persistent leakage can be distressing, contribute to other gynecologic problems, and affect the quality of life.

The primary risk factor for stress incontinence is childbirth and pregnancy. In reproductive-aged women, more than 50 percent of the cases of urinary incontinence can be attributed to pregnancy and childbirth. Women who deliver vaginally are 3 times more likely to develop incontinence.[4] Pregnancy itself is a risk factor, but the problem can be exacerbated when the pelvic floor is damaged because of birth. Other risk factors include age, obesity, menopause, pelvic injury, genetic or congenital issues, chronic cough, and chronic constipation.

In continent women, the muscles of the urethra and pelvic floor work in coordination to store urine and evacuate at an appropriate time. Childbirth and other factors that damage the nerves and muscles could result in weakness and dysfunction. The muscles of the urethra and pelvic floor become too weak and cannot prevent the forceful expulsion of urine that occurs with a hard cough or sudden sneeze. In some cases, the nerve damage makes it difficult for the bladder to sense when it is full or can prevent the bladder from sending the correct message to the brain. Uninhibited bladder contractions may lead to unplanned bladder emptying.

Damage caused during childbirth usually improves over time, and often resolves within one year after giving birth. Most women report some degree of incontinence during pregnancy that also resolves after birth. The muscles and nerves either recover completely or learn to compensate.

Recurrent births, age, and other factors may inflict further damage on the muscles, and they then may cross the threshold where compensation is no longer possible and the incontinence becomes a persistent problem that gradually worsens. Pelvic muscle exercises before pregnancy, during pregnancy, and after delivery has been shown to help minimize this problem; however, this practice has not been incorporated as routine recommendation of health care providers.

Conservative Treatment of Stress Urinary Incontinence

Most women will experience mild symptoms of stress urinary incontinence and can take advantage of conservative treatment options. Depending on the severity of the symptoms, a woman can initiate some of this on her own or complete an evaluation by a qualified provider to confirm the diagnosis.

The initial evaluation will consist of a thorough history and physical examination, including a pelvic examination and an assessment of pelvic muscle strength. It is important to have a urinalysis and a urine culture as conditions like a urinary tract infection can present with leakage. More detailed testing, such as the completion of a bladder diary, assessment of post-void residual and urodynamics, may be recommended. These can help to distinguish between the different types of incontinence, determine the severity of the problem and help the doctor make appropriate treatment recommendations.

Behavioral therapy and physiotherapy are the most common suggestions. Behavioral therapy involves developing coping mechanisms and minimizing opportunities for leakage. Examples include pre-urge voiding to avoid developing urgency or voiding before exercise to keep the bladder volume low, as some women will only leak with a full bladder. Weight loss is another method. Women who are obese and overweight may note a significant improvement in their leakage as they lose body fat.

Physiotherapy involves strengthening the muscles of the pelvic floor. This involves doing the traditional kegel exercises, which involve squeezing the pelvic floor muscles and holding the squeeze for a set period and doing a certain number of repetitions. Like lifting weights, the muscles become stronger over time with increased repetition and endurance. Sometimes the exercises are not easy to perform and electrical stimulation and/or biofeedback helps with identifying, isolating, and activating the muscles. Pelvic muscles exercises are about 50 to 60 percent effective in the treatment of stress urinary incontinence.[5]

Devices such as pessaries and urethra plugs have been developed to prevent leakage. They work by obstructing the urethra, preventing urine from passing during a stressful event. These are not widely popular due to the inconvenience and possible discomfort of inserting and wearing a device, but may be valuable in certain select situation, such as use during exercise only. Medications have been researched for stress incontinence, but currently only one called duloxetine has been shown to provide some degree of improvement. There are some challenges with taking this medication, including limited availability of the drug.

Conservative therapy should be considered to manage stress urinary incontinence, especially in women who have only mild symptoms. Surgery is certainly more effective, but has risks that can only be justified in women whose symptoms are seriously negatively affecting their lives.

Surgical Treatment

Minimally invasive procedures are currently the ideal approach for modern incontinence care. In the past, retropubic urethropexy surgeries like the Burch or MMK procedure were considered the "gold standard." In these procedures, the tissue on either side of the urethra is sewn to the pubic bone providing better support. These procedures require an incision on the abdomen. These were replaced by bladder neck suspensions such as the Stamey procedure and the bladder neck slings which also provide support to the urethra but the surgery is done through the vagina making them less invasive than the retropubic urethropexy with comparable outcomes. Other procedures include periurethral injections, which offer some improvement but are far from the cure offered by the slings and the retropubic urethropexies.

Currently the most popular and effective surgical treatment is the mid-urethra sling, which is a minimally invasive procedure that is highly effective and has a low risk of complications. This procedure utilizes smaller incisions and a strip of synthetic mesh to support the urethra. The success rate ranges from 80 to 90 percent, comparable to the Burch procedure, but with many more advantages. This procedure was first described in 1993 and has rapidly become the surgery of choice for female stress incontinence. The ease of the procedure and low complication rate has made it possible for many more women to achieve a cure. By 2006, 1 out of every 1,000 women in the U.S. were taking advantage of the availability of anti-incontinence surgery.

Since its introduction as the tension-free vaginal tape (TVT), the mid-urethral sling has undergone several improvements. Currently this sling is available in 3 different approaches: the retropubic, the transobturator, and the single incision sling. Each has its advantages and disadvantages and surgeons have their personal preferences. The cure rate for the retropubic version is 85 to 92 percent, while the cure rate for the transobturator approach is 73 to 81 percent. The complication rates tend to be a bit higher with the retropubic approach, which is why the transobturator approach is appealing. The single incision sling is relatively new and has a reported 1-year success rate of 76 percent.[6]

Stress incontinence can be cured or improved. Effective surgeries are available and can be done via minimally invasive techniques. The most important step is to select the right provider and be clear on the options. Surgery should only be undertaken if the severity of the symptoms warrants the surgical risks. It is prudent to first consider conservative therapy, especially if the symptoms are mild.

Sling Complications

The retropubic mid-urethra sling, also called the transvaginal tape (TVT), was the first in its class. They all use a polypropylene (a plastic polymer) mesh strip, which is incorporated into the peri-urethra tissue. In theory, this should provide a permanent fix of the problem. The cure rate for this sling is reported at 85 to 92 percent at 5 years. Issues associated with this sling include a 34 percent urinary tract infection rate at 3 months, a reported voiding dysfunction (incomplete or difficult voiding) rate of 20 to 47 percent, and a 25 percent risk of urinary urgency. Other more severe complications include bladder injury up to 7 percent, mesh erosion as high as 2.5 percent and inability to void at 3 months in 3 percent. Rare but serious complications also include intestinal and vascular injury requiring blood transfusion, additional surgery, and even death.[7]

The transobturator mid-urethra sling was developed to avoid the more serious complications seen in the retropubic mid-urethra sling. Its insertion site is farther away from the bladder and the vital organs in the pelvis. The cure rates are reported 73 to 81 percent, while the risk of voiding dysfunction is significantly lower at less than 11 percent. The urinary tract infection (6.4 percent) and bladder injury rates (less 1 percent) are also much less. The mesh erosion rate is about the same, while there is a much higher rate of groin or leg pain, which occurs in 12 to 16 percent of the cases. As with the retropubic sling the incidence of vascular and intestinal injury are rare.

The single incision slings, also called mini-slings, were developed to make the procedure even easier and with even fewer complications. Less mesh is used and only a single incision is required to insert the sling. The procedure can even be performed in the office setting with local anesthesia. This is a relatively new procedure so long term data about effectiveness is limited. The 12-month data suggests a cure rate of about 76 percent with voiding dysfunction occurring less than 10 percent of the time. The rate of mesh extrusion/exposure is about the same as the other slings.

Each sling has its pros and cons. The idea is to select the most appropriate procedure to minimize the risk of complications but maximize the chance of success. This is where an experienced surgeon comes in handy. It is easy to decide to do the surgery and equally easy to perform any of these procedures. The key is to have a provider who selects the right procedure the first time and who can manage any complication that may arise. Sling outcomes can be unpredictable, so it is best to choose a surgeon who has the proper training and experience.

Managing Sling Complications

The mid-urethra sling is the most popular procedure for stress incontinence and its wide availability has made it possible for many women to be cured. Not all surgeries are successful, and even in those that are can have some bumps in the road. So, what happens if you experience a sling complications?

First, it is important to remember that the chance of success is high, so most women undergoing surgery will not have any problems. The most common problems after sling surgery include the inability to void completely, a urinary tract infection, failure of the procedure, mesh erosion or exposure, or subsequent voiding dysfunction. These can be managed with minimal long-term effects.

The possibility of difficulty voiding should have been discussed before the surgery. This happens. Some women can't void at all while others can only void partially. This usually resolves in a week or two, but you should be prepared to either perform intermittent self-catherization or go home with a catheter in place to continuously drain the bladder. If the issue has not resolved in three weeks at the most, your surgeon can take you back to the surgical suite to loosen the sling. If the incomplete voiding problem persists for much longer the sling may need to be cut. Some women experience this incomplete voiding months and years after the procedure and removal of the sling is also a possibility.

Ideally, you will have a 100 percent cure after the sling surgery; however, this doesn't always occur. As much as 75 percent or more improvement can certainly be considered a success, especially if you have gone from leaking a lot to only losing a few drops. If, however, there is no perceptible improvement, let your doctor know as soon as possible. There is a way to go back to surgery to attempt some type of tightening, but the window of opportunity is narrow.

Urinary tract infections are common after bladder procedures, and are usually treated with oral antibiotics. Voiding dysfunction includes urinary frequency, urgency, and even urge incontinence, and this is a potential risk of bladder surgery that cannot be avoided. If the dysfunction involves incomplete emptying, then cutting or removing the sling is an option. Finally, mesh erosions or exposure into the vagina are usually managed by use of estrogen cream in postmenopausal women or cutting and burying the exposed mesh. Major complications are rare, but are managed in conjunction with the appropriate clinical expert based on the scenario.

Sling surgery is an excellent option for those who suffer from stress urinary incontinence that has not responded to conservative measures. No treatment is without its risks. Take the time to do the due diligence in choosing your provider and partner with them to make sure you fully understand the treatment recommendations, the planned procedure, the potential complications, and risks, as well as the postsurgical expectations.

Pelvic Organ Prolapse

Pelvic organ prolapse includes uterine prolapse, cystocele, rectocele, enterocele, and vaginal vault prolapse. When uterine supports become weak, the uterus gradually drops into the vagina. The cervix can be felt or seen dropping through the vaginal opening. A cystocele occurs when the vaginal wall that rests underneath the bladder starts to drop down. Its supports have also become weak, and as this wall drops down and through the vagina the bladder will follow. This occurs because the vaginal wall is part of the bladder's support structure. A rectocele occurs when the vaginal wall that rests on top of the rectum becomes weak and bulges up into the vaginal lumen and sometimes out through the opening. The rectal wall will subsequently follow because this vaginal wall is part of the support structure for the rectum. An enterocele occurs when a weakness develops in the upper vaginal wall just underneath the cervix. Some loops of intestine can fall behind the vaginal wall in this area, causing a bulge in the vagina. Vaginal vault prolapse occurs in women who have had a hysterectomy when all the vaginal walls are poorly supported. As a result, the vagina can gradually fall down, essentially "turning inside out" like a sock.

Prolapse occurs when the structures that support the uterus and vagina are damaged. The support structures include the pelvic floor muscles, connective tissue, and ligaments all designed to keep the vagina closed and attached to the pelvic sidewall, holding the internal organs in place. The nerves are vital components to this support system that communicate with the muscles so they can function properly. The most common factor contributing to the development of prolapse is vaginal childbirth. During delivery, the nerves can be stretched and connective tissue torn. The pelvic muscles can also be damaged either directly or because of nerve damage. If the nerves are damaged they cannot communicate with the muscles. These muscles will then atrophy and grow weak from disuse. Damage to these support structures can also occur because of pelvic surgery, trauma to the pelvis, and other conditions that might affect the lumbar and sacral regions of the spinal cord.

Symptoms of uterine prolapse include feeling a bulge, pelvic pressure, back pain and discomfort, or even pain with intercourse. A cystocele can present with a bulge, frequency and urgency of urination, difficulty urinating, and recurrent urinary tract infections. Symptoms of a rectocele also include a bulge, difficulty with intercourse and difficulty having bowel movements. Some women may need to press on the vagina to empty their rectum. An enterocele and vaginal vault prolapse usually present with a notable bulge in the vagina, pelvic pressure and pain, and problems with intercourse.

Treatments for prolapse are available and may include pelvic floor muscle rehabilitation, wearing a supportive device called a pessary or surgery. A thorough evaluation is required to make the correct diagnosis and appropriate recommendations for treatment. It is important to be evaluated by an experienced gynecologic surgeon. Urogynecologists are gynecologic surgeons who have special training in this area.

Even though surgery is generally effective, prevention is the key. Research is ongoing to identify better measures to prevent the development of this problem. Advancements in the treatment and prevention of this problem will eventually be limited by the availability of funds for such research.

Overactive Bladder

Are you constantly going to the bathroom? Do you know the location of every bathroom in the mall? Do you experience a sudden powerful urge to urinate as soon as you put the key in your front door or right when you get to the bathroom?

If you answered yes to any of these questions, then you are 1 of the 30 million people who suffer from a condition called "overactive bladder." Overactive bladder (OAB) is a syndrome that includes the symptoms of urinary frequency, urgency, and sometimes urge incontinence. It is normal to void 7 to 8 times during the day and get up no more than twice after going to sleep at night. Urinating more than this is abnormal. Urgency is the sudden compelling desire to void that cannot be ignored. For some women, this is associated with urinary leakage (or wetting themselves); this is urge incontinence.

Overactive bladder is not a life-threatening condition, but it is a life altering one. This problem has financial, social, and health implications. Women who suffer from this condition typically use protective pads, which can be expensive. Imagine the cost if one is changing pads several times a day. Going to the bathroom frequently and needing to get there in a hurry can affect one's work and social life. If someone is constantly in the bathroom, they can't be a productive worker. Many women elect to stay closer to home to avoid embarrassing leakage episodes. Thus, they travel less and have less social interactions. This can lead to feelings of isolation and depression. This problem is also associated with an increased risk of falls, which in an older person could lead to fractures and an increased risk of morbidity and even death.

Overactive Bladder Treatment

Treatment options are available, but despite this only a small percentage of individuals seek care or are treated. This is due to a lack of knowledge of treatment availability on the patients' part and a lack of knowledge of management options on the part of the healthcare provider. Seeking care with an urogynecologist (a specialist in Female Pelvic Medicine) or a urologist is appropriate if the primary care physician lacks experience in treating this condition.

The initial evaluation should focus on identifying easily treated and reversible conditions such as a urinary tract infection. Once the diagnosis of overactive bladder is made, treatments can be discussed. Some women have improvement with dietary changes. Eliminating food and beverages that irritate the bladder can provide significant improvement. These items include coffee (even decaffeinated), tea, sodas (even diet), citrus fruits, and artificial sweeteners. Postmenopausal women may experience improvement with the administration of vaginal estrogen. Pelvic floor muscle exercises (kegels) and bladder retraining are effective when done appropriately. Most women need to do this under the supervision of a Pelvic Floor Physical Therapist or a Nurse Continence Specialist. In addition, these professionals can provide other options, including electrical stimulation.

Medications are also available. They fall into the category of anticholingeric or antimuscarinic agents, which work by blocking specific receptors in the bladder to prevent binding of acetylcholine, a neurotransmitter that causes the bladder to contract. The result is fewer episodes of urge incontinence and an improvement in the symptoms of frequency and urgency. These medications are effective but can have side effects. They can bind to receptors in other parts of the body leading to dry eyes, dry mouth, and constipation. In addition, they can affect cognitive function. Finally, they are not recommended for people who have difficulty with bladder emptying, gastric emptying, severe constipation, or narrowed angle glaucoma. These medications include Oxybutynin, Tolterodine, Darifenacin, Trospium, Solifenacin and others.

Medications are not perfect but can be very effective in many individuals. Sacral nerve stimulation (Interstim) is an alternative in cases where conservative therapy has failed or when medications are not an option. This procedure stimulates one of the sacral nerves, usually the S3 nerve, leading to improvement in frequency, urgency, and urge incontinence. The advantage of this procedure is that one can test it out before having it placed permanently. It has been a godsend to many suffering individuals. Another nerve stimulation procedure, called percutaneous tibial nerve stimulation (Urgent PC) is an in-office weekly treatment that also improves the symptoms of overactive bladder.

The symptoms of urinary frequency, urgency, and urge incontinence can be life-altering. Treatment options are available and the variety is such that most women should be able to find one that meets her needs. You don't have to let your bladder problems ruin your life.

Fecal Incontinence

This is the involuntary loss of feces. Anal incontinence, a term sometimes used interchangeably, is the involuntary loss of flatus as well as stool. This is a potentially distressing problem affecting around 15 percent of women.[1-3] The major contributor to this problem is childbirth, and the number one factor is damage to the anal sphincter at the time of delivery. A third- or fourth-degree laceration, also referred to as obstetric anal sphincter injury (OASI), occurs in up to 6 percent of women after birth, and of those who experience this injury, up to 24 percent will develop anal incontinence.

Although not widely discussed, this is a common problem and there are ways to prevent and treat it. Prevention entails avoiding labor-related factors that contribute to OASI. Forceps use is one of these factors; however, it is important to remember that there are some benefits to forceps use as well. It is important to discuss this with your obstetrician if you are pregnant. If you had an OASI in a previous delivery, then a Cesarean section for subsequent deliveries should be considered.

If you are experiencing symptoms of anal incontinence and would like help, then you should seek the advice of a urogynecologist or a colorectal surgeon. You can find a provider at <u>augs.org</u> or <u>fascrs.org</u>.

THE BOTTOM LINE

- Vaginal birth is the primary cause of pelvic floor problems in women, but there are other factors.
- Pelvic floor problems include prolapse, incontinence of urine or stool, and difficulty controlling the bladder.
- These problems are not life-threatening and treatment should be decided based on the severity of symptoms.

Chapter 11

Other Health Challenges

Gynecologists recognize a woman's well-being can be significantly affected by common health conditions such as hypertension, diabetes, heart disease, and cerebrovascular disease. These problems are so common that physicians, no matter their specialty, are obligated to be on the lookout for signs or symptoms in their patients. Most gynecologists consider themselves to be the primary care provider for women and will screen their patients for these problems and educate them on their hazards. This chapter will review these common medical problems.

Hypertension

Brianna is here for her routine gynecologic examination. I noted that her blood pressure was 160/100. On reviewing her records her blood pressure had been high at the last visit and I had referred her to an internist. "Did you see the internist I referred you to last year?" I ask. She gives a big sigh and says, "Yes, I did, and he placed me on a medication but I stopped taking it after a few weeks because I didn't like the way it made me feel. I felt better off the medications so I didn't go back." I take the time to explain to Brianna that hypertension doesn't cause symptoms until it's too late to save vital organs from damage. I call one of my Internal Medicine colleagues and he agrees to see her the same day.

What is hypertension?

Hypertension, or high blood pressure, occurs when the blood vessels of the arterial system become constricted, forcing the heart to work harder to pump the blood to the tissues of the body. This pressure is determined when the blood pressure is measured. Hypertension is present when the pressure is consistently greater than 140/90.

A survey done between 1999 and 2008 reported that 29 percent of adults suffer from high blood pressure. This means approximately 60 million people or more are affected. It's no surprise then that managing high blood pressure is the most common reason for doctor visits among non-pregnant adults in the U.S.[1]

Essential hypertension is the most common type of high blood pressure. While the cause is unclear, there are many possible theories. One theory concerns an increase in the activity of the nerves that control the blood vessels, causing the arteries to be more contracted. This leads to higher pressures. Another theory suggests that it's an increase in the circulating amounts of certain hormones that also affect the activity of the vessels. Other theories suggest a genetic role and/or a decrease in the kidney cell mass, which plays a role in blood pressure control. Obviously much more research is needed to identify more specific causes.

Secondary hypertension is high blood pressure caused by another medical condition. Kidney problems, specifically renal artery stenosis, the narrowing of the major artery supplying the kidney, are a major cause for increased blood pressure. Obstruction of the ureter, the duct that passes urine from the kidney to the bladder, and damage to the kidney from diseases such as diabetes and lupus are other examples. It is important to identify these causes to avoid subsequent renal failure. In addition, treating these problems could potentially resolve the hypertension. High blood pressure may also be triggered by an overproduction of certain substances that affect the arteries. Examples include tumors that produce adrenaline and over-active adrenal or thyroid glands. Finally, medications such as birth control pills and steroids can contribute to the development of hypertension.

Hypertension in its early stages doesn't cause any noticeable symptoms. Many people can have high blood pressure for many years and not have any noticeable symptoms. If the pressure becomes excessively high (>200/100) then symptoms such as headaches, blurred vision, and confusion can occur. This is called "malignant hypertension" and could result in stroke, rupture of an aneurysm, and a heart attack. Long-term uncontrolled hypertension can lead to organ damage, too. If the heart must work harder to pump blood, it is likely to fail over time. Heart failure results in disability, diminished quality of life, and premature death. Chronic uncontrolled hypertension can also lead to renal failure and a possible need for dialysis, visual impairment and possible blindness, and other organ damage.

Diagnosing and treating hypertension is crucial in identifying and preventing potentially life-threatening problems. Screening is easy; all it takes is a visit to your doctor.

How is blood pressure classified?

Blood pressure measurements are typically written with the systolic pressure on top and the diastolic pressure on the bottom; for example, 120 over 80. The systolic pressure is the pressure in the arteries measured at the time of the heart contraction (heart beat) and the diastolic at the time of heart relaxation or between beats when the heart is refilling with blood.

Normal blood pressure is a systolic of less than 120 and a diastolic pressure less than 80. Pre-hypertension is a blood pressure of 120 to 139 over 80 to 89. Stage 1 hypertension occurs when the blood pressure is 140 to 159 over 90 to 99 while Stage 2 occurs when the pressure is 160 over 100 or higher. This classification is helpful in determining treatment recommendations.

Why is hypertension a big deal?

Untreated, long standing hypertension can lead to many problems. When the heart works harder to pump blood through the arteries, it will hypertrophy (become enlarged) over time, eventually failing. An enlarged heart is also prone to developing abnormal rhythms, which could result in sudden death. Hypertension may lead to myocardial infarction (MI), also known as heart attack, in those with coronary artery disease. It can lead to stroke and kidney failure. These consequences are even more likely to occur in the setting of other problems, such as diabetes or atherosclerosis (hardening of the arteries).

Who gets hypertension?

Age is the major risk factor in developing hypertension. The older we get, the more likely we are to develop high blood pressure. It is present in most people over 65 years of age. Race is another major risk factor; for example, it is more prevalent in African Americans. Other factors include obesity, sedentary lifestyle, family history, elevated blood lipids, excessive salt intake, and excessive alcohol use.

Why isn't everyone treated?

Many people have heard of high blood pressure or at least know of someone being treated for it, but not many truly understand the potentially grave consequences of leaving it untreated or inadequately treated. One study estimated that 50 percent of those treated are not adequately controlled.[3] The numbers of those who are untreated is unclear, but estimates indicate a very high number.

There are many reasons why this is occurring. Obviously, there is a lack of understanding about the consequences of not diagnosing and treating high blood pressure. For many, the absence of symptoms leads to complacency, but significant problems may occur. This is where health education and literacy may play a role. Some of the people who are not treated have poor access to health care and are unable to pay for the required medication.

How is hypertension diagnosed?

Hypertension is diagnosed by documenting the elevated pressure at random times over a period of several weeks, often during a series of 3 to 6 doctor visits. The other option is for a patient to check blood pressure at home using a blood pressure monitor that can be purchased in a pharmacy or online. The pressure should be checked both at stress-free times and at random times during the day to simulate normal life. If necessary, 24-hour monitoring by a medical professional at a medical facility can be done. The information gathered while doing this can help a physician devise an appropriate treatment plan. If the blood pressure is in the pre-hypertension range or at Stage 1, then there is time to institute lifestyle changes. If the blood pressure is greater than 160 over 100, urgent treatment is required. This is described as hypertension urgency. Malignant hypertension exists when the blood pressure is in the severe range and the patient has symptoms such as headaches and confusion. This usually requires admission to the hospital for immediate control.

Once hypertension is diagnosed, further evaluation is recommended. The goal is to determine the possible cause of the elevated blood pressure and the level of organ damage that may have been sustained prior to diagnosis.

The evaluation should first consist of a thorough history and physical examination. The urine is analyzed for the presence of protein, which may indicate kidney damage. Blood work is also drawn to evaluate kidney function and to search for other medical problems, such as diabetes and elevated cholesterol. An electrocardiogram (ECG) is done to evaluate the condition of the heart. It may reveal evidence of heart failure, abnormal rhythm, or an unrecognized heart attack. Another test may include a detailed eye examination looking for retinal damage. Other scans or special tests may be ordered to look for arterial aneurysms and kidney function.

Early detection and treatment of hypertension could save your life. It is important for every adult to have his or her blood pressure monitored on a regular basis. This is routinely done at all doctor's visits. You should know what your blood pressure is and, if it is higher than it should be, follow your doctor's advice for further monitoring or evaluation. Hypertension prevention may be, for many, as simple as exercising on a regular basis and controlling your weight.

Treating Hypertension

Lifestyle changes such as weight loss, regular aerobic exercise, and restricting the amount of salt in your diet are effective in treating mild hypertension and helpful in managing high blood pressure in those who also require medication.

If you have been diagnosed with high blood pressure, take that warning seriously. Those who have hypertension are at risk of developing heart failure, heart attack, and stroke. The risks of these events are increased if you also have elevated lipids, like cholesterol, and diabetes. If you have these conditions, controlling them all is crucial to prevent heart disease and other complications. We all must die of something, but the goal is to maintain a good quality of life for as long as possible. Controlling hypertension allows you to achieve this goal.

Medications Used to Treat Hypertension

All the medications used to treat hypertension are equally effective, with a response rate of 30 to 50 percent. There is, however, individual variability in response and tolerance of any given medication. In general, it is the reduction in blood pressure that decreases the risk of complications and not the actual medication itself. There are certain groups that tend to do better with one category versus the other. For instance, the elderly and African Americans tend to respond better to thiazide diuretics or calcium channel blockers while younger people seem to do better with angiotensin converting enzyme (ACE) inhibitors and angiotensin II receptor blockers (ARB).

Thiazide diuretics such as hydrochlorothiazide and chlorthalidone are typically used as an initial treatment. They work by decreasing the sodium reabsorption in the nephrons (absorption unit of the kidney). This increases the sodium in the urine, thereby increasing the water loss. The dose of the medication is 12.5 to 100 mg daily. Chlorthalidone is preferred for many reasons, including a lower effective dose. Side effects and complications include glucose intolerance, low potassium, increased uric acid, and low magnesium. As with most medications, using the lowest effective dose tends to minimize intolerable side effects.

Angiotensin converting enzyme (ACE) inhibitors and angiotensin II receptor blockers (ARB) decrease or block the substance angiotensin, a vasoconstrictor chemical that in turn raises the blood pressure. Commonly used ones include enalapril, lisinopril, captopril, valsartan, telmisartan, and losartan, though there are many others. These medications are generally well tolerated but have the common side effects of cough and swelling. They can cause birth defects and should not be taken by pregnant women. This category of hypertensive medications is especially indicated when someone also has a history of heart failure, a prior heart attack, chronic kidney disease, or diabetes mellitus.

Calcium channel blockers (CCB) inhibit the calcium channels in cells. There are two types: the dihydropyridines, which cause vasodilation but don't affect the vascular permeability, and the non-dihydropyridines, which also decrease vascular permeability and affect myocardial contractility and conduction. Commonly used medications in this category include diltiazem, verapamil, amlodipine, and nifedipine. Common side effects include headache, dizziness, flushing, and swelling. These medications also are used sometimes to control heart arrhythmias.

Beta-blockers are rarely used as a first line agent in the treatment of high blood pressure. They work by blocking the effect of epinephrine, thus slowing the heart rate and causing vasodilation. They tend to be useful in the management of arrhythmias, heart failure, and the control of blood pressure after a heart attack. Common side effects include nausea, vomiting, diarrhea, dizziness, headache, and glucose intolerance.

In many cases a single agent isn't effective and the addition of a second drug may be required to get ideal blood pressure control. In this scenario, drugs from different categories are used. Common combinations include diuretics with CCB or diuretics with ACE/ARB, and even CCB with ACE/ARB. This is such a common practice that these combination medications have been manufactured and can be prescribed in a single pill.

If you take medications to control your blood pressure, I suggest you become knowledgeable about the medication. You should know the dosage, the brand and generic name, how the pill looks, and expected side effects. Always take the medication as prescribed and follow up with your doctor if you have any problems. When the medication is issued by the pharmacy, always review the name and dosage to confirm it is what your doctor prescribed. If the appearance of the drug is different than you expected, return to the pharmacist and ask questions. Make sure the answer is acceptable to you. Medication errors are common and you should make sure you or family members are receiving the right drugs.

Diabetes

I took care of Yvonne during her last pregnancy 5 years ago, but hadn't seen her since. She showed me pictures of her family and told me what she had been up to. "Dr. Howard, don't scold me but I haven't seen a doctor since my delivery. But I remembered what you told me, 'To take care of your family, you need to take care of yourself.' So, I'm here to get a complete checkup." I gave her a hug and said, "I'm glad you came back." On reviewing her records, I find that she had gestational diabetes during her last pregnancy so in addition to the routine gynecologic test I also ordered a glucose tolerance test. The test was abnormal and I referred her to an internist to manage her newly diagnosed Type 2 diabetes mellitus.

Diabetes is a popular health topic, claiming the attention of the media and medical experts. There are different types of diabetes, but the most common one is Type 2, often described as adult onset diabetes mellitus. Much of the focus of health campaigns refers to this type. Type 2 diabetes mellitus (T2DM) has become more prevalent and is associated with many other life-threatening conditions. But what is it?

Our body converts carbohydrates into glucose, a kind of sugar. Insulin is required to transport that glucose into the cells so it can be used or stored for energy. Type 2 diabetes mellitus is a condition wherein there is a problem with the utilization of glucose and function of insulin. Signs of this condition include a higher than normal blood glucose level, a condition called hyperglycemia. Resistance to the effects of insulin or impaired insulin secretion is also found. A diagnosis is made when there is evidence of persistent hyperglycemia and insulin resistance is confirmed over time.

Glucose levels that are consistently elevated contribute to a vicious cycle because the elevated glucose can harm the cells in the pancreas responsible for secreting insulin. This leads to further insulin resistance and impaired secretion, which subsequently causes higher levels of blood glucose. Control of blood glucose levels is needed to break the cycle and to prevent further damage to the pancreas.

The development of diabetes is a complex process and can't be attributed to one cause. A genetic susceptibility to insulin problems has been identified and multiple genes are involved. It is also clear that obesity is a major contributor to the onset of this problem, but the degree of excessive weight, which may trigger the problem, varies in individuals. Every obese person does not develop diabetes and not everyone with diabetes mellitus is overweight. However, significant weight loss in individuals with diabetes can lead to a cure of the diabetes. Other contributors include low physical activity and diet. Increased physical activity and appropriate diet improves diabetes.

Elevated glucose levels alone are not of concern, but if persistent over a long period can have serious consequences. Long term and uncontrolled diabetes can lead to heart attack, kidney failure, strokes, vision loss, and vascular compromise causing loss of extremities. Diabetes prevention and management can save your life.

Problem of Diabetes

Type 2 diabetes affects approximately 14 percent of people in the U.S. and 38% have pre-diabetes. It is estimated that 36 percent of these people are unaware they have the condition.[6] The economic implications are extensive as this problem accounts for a significant percentage of U.S. healthcare expenditures. Uncontrolled diabetes causes extensive vascular damage leading to heart attack, stroke, kidney failure, amputation, and blindness.

Diabetes in children, primarily attributed to obesity, has increased. The earlier the onset of diabetes, the more likely an individual will suffer from the above problems and have premature death. In 2001, the prevalence of Type 2 diabetes in children was about 3 percent. The numbers affected increased to 4.6 percent in 2009. Overall there has been a 30 percent increase in Type 2 diabetes in children.[8] This is a public health crisis.

A diet that is high in sugar, which often leads to weight gain and possibly obesity, can contribute to further problems with glucose control. There is also a genetic predisposition to diabetes. Some individuals are more prone to developing these problems, and the triggers are many. Some will eventually develop it as they age, while others spark the condition with poor eating habits, alcohol use, and minimal activity.

The western diet of fast foods, eating for entertainment, and consuming excessive calories is killing us. In addition, the lifestyle of little to no physical activity is adding fuel to the fire. Diet and exercise habits are established in childhood. Our children are being taught bad habits and these are difficult to break as adults.

The solution is simple for many. A nutritious diet, regular physical activity, and weight management can ward off diabetes in many, especially children. Even those with a genetic predisposition to diabetes can benefit. A healthy diet, weight control, and regular exercise help improve glucose control in those with diabetes. Prevention, however, is the ideal and this should be the target for our children. In individuals with the condition, these activities are beneficial and can help those affected live a long and healthy life.

<u>Who gets type 2 diabetes?</u>

People who develop type 2 diabetes have certain factors in common, including age, being overweight, a family history of the disease, and are part of certain ethnic or racial groups who are more likely to get the disease.

Adults over 45 years of age have a greater risk of developing diabetes. Over 39 percent of people with T2DM have at least one parent with diabetes.[9] T2DM is 2 to 6 times more prevalent in African Americans, Native Americans, and Hispanic Americans than in white Americans. Those with a body mass index (BMI) of more than 25 are at higher risk. Morbidly obese individuals (BMI more than 40) with T2DM who lose a significant amount of weight often can be cured of this condition. This is best illustrated in the bariatric surgery population where the majority of individuals no longer require treatment of their diabetes after the surgery.

Most people who develop type 2 diabetes have a genetic predisposition. There appears to be a defect in the genes involved in insulin secretion. The defects are likely multiple, and some are located at the level of insulin synthesis while others are in the development of the beta cells (cells that make insulin). This supports family history as a risk factor for the disease.

Diabetes contributes to significant medical problems that can lead to premature death. In the long term, uncontrolled diabetes causes vascular damage over time. This damage can manifest itself as circulatory problems causing leg pain, especially with activity. This is called claudication. This poor circulation can also lead to foot ulcers and, if unchecked, can lead to a need for amputation. The same type of vascular damage can cause a heart attack or stroke, which could result in immediate death or disability. The kidneys can be damaged, resulting in renal failure over time and the need for dialysis. The vessels in the eye are also affected, causing retinopathy, which can lead to a decrease in vision and even loss of sight.

The consequences of diabetes are many, and it is important for you to know if you are at risk. There is much that can be done to prevent T2DM. Regular exercise, weight management, and an appropriate diet are the keys. It requires discipline to follow these regimens, but the payoff is certainly worth it.

Screening for Diabetes

It is impossible to screen everyone, so the focus of early diagnosis should be on those at risk. The American Diabetes Association (ADA) recommends screening every 3 years for everyone over the age of 45. Other screening should be done based on the presence of risk factors and is at the discretion of the doctor. Obesity, family history, and being a member of a high-risk group are factors that should drive earlier screening.

Available screening tests include a fasting serum (blood) glucose level, a 2-hour glucose tolerance test, or a hemoglobin A1C. The fasting glucose level is checked after 8 to 16 hours without food or drink. The value is less than 100 mg/dl in healthy individuals. If it is 100 to 125 then the person is considered to have pre-diabetes, and if it's 126 or greater then diabetes is present. The values should be repeated to confirm the diagnosis.

The 2-hour glucose tolerance test requires checking a fasting serum glucose, followed by the consumption of 75 grams of glucose. The serum glucose level is then measured again 1 hour and 2 hours later. The fasting values are the same as above. The 2-hour result should be less than 140. They are described as having impaired glucose tolerance when the value is between 140 and 200 and diabetes when it is more than 200. A similar test is done during pregnancy with different cut-off values.

The hemoglobin (hgb) A1C test, also referred to as glycosylated hemoglobin or A1C test, is used to diagnose both types of diabetes. It measures the percentage of hemoglobin that is coated in sugar. The values reflect the average blood sugar (glucose) levels for the past 2 to 3 months. Normal individuals have values less than 5.7 percent, while pre-diabetes is present when the value is 5.7 to 6.4 percent, and 6.5 percent and greater is confirmation of diabetes.

If you or any family member has symptoms or risk factors for diabetes, a screening test is highly recommended. Tests with abnormal values can be repeated to confirm accuracy. If your values reflect pre-diabetes, then you can initiate lifestyle changes that can prevent or prolong the onset of diabetes. If you are diagnosed with diabetes, then treatment is available to manage the condition before it causes irreversible damage. You have the power to prevent long-term problems. If you are at risk, get screened.

Treating Diabetes

Some people will develop T2DM despite lifestyle intervention. Medications are available to treat diabetes. These oral agents are designed to help control the serum glucose levels. The most popular is metformin. It is well studied, helps with modest weight loss, and has minimal side effects. In a diabetes prevention program, individuals who took metformin reduced their risk of developing diabetes by 31 percent. Other agents are also available and can be used in combination with metformin. For those whose diabetes is difficult to control, insulin maybe needed. Remember, the goal of treatment is to make sure the serum glucose levels remain in a normal range all the time. This is the way to prevent vascular damage.

If you have been diagnosed with diabetes, your doctor should not only treat you for the diabetes but also look for evidence of vascular damage. Tests should be done to make sure the vital organs are not showing any ill-effects from chronic hyperglycemia. An electrocardiogram can evaluate the heart while blood and urine tests can check kidney function. An eye examination, specifically looking at the vessels of the retina, can see if there is early damage. Your doctor may recommend an in-depth examination of your feet by a podiatrist.

There are other conditions that can work in concert with diabetes to cause problems. If you have elevated cholesterol (hyperlipidemia) and/or hypertension, these conditions should be treated to prevent organ damage. If you smoke, you should quit as this is extremely toxic to the body's blood vessels. Smoking, hyperlipidemia, and hypertension can cause heart disease and stroke alone; imagine what damage can occur when these are present along with diabetes.

Type 2 diabetes mellitus is a common problem, but it can be managed to prevent chronic organ damage and premature death. You can start by developing healthy habits, such as regular exercise and a proper diet. Stop smoking and lose weight. If you have risk factors or symptoms, see a doctor and ask about diabetes screening. Take control of your health and do what is needed so you can increase your chance of living a healthy life.

Heart Attack and Stroke

I noticed Stella rubbing her left arm as she paused while emptying the trash. She seemed to be moving slower than usual. She has worked as a custodian on the gynecology unit for years and is a fast, efficient worker. "Are you okay?" I paused and gave her a close look. She doesn't look well and tells me that she has been experiencing intermittent numbness in her left arm and some shortness of breath. These symptoms are concerning for a heart attack or stroke, so I insisted that she have a seat so one of the nurses could take her blood pressure. It was alarmingly high, so we placed her in a wheelchair and took her straight to the emergency department. We didn't stop at the reception desk, despite being scolded by the receptionist, but took her straight back and demanded that she be assessed right away. Turns out she was having a myocardial infarction and was rushed to the cardiac suite for an immediate heart catheterization.

Understanding the Heart

Heart disease is the number one cause of death in the U.S., and the world! Most people know this but many are not clear on how the heart works and why it is at risk for damage.

To understand heart disease, you must first understand the heart. The heart is a muscle about the size of a fist. It is in the thoracic cavity between the lungs. It contains 4 chambers, which are separated by walls, called septa, and structures like doors, called valves, which control the flow of blood from one chamber to the next. The primary goal of the heart is to pump blood through the body. The blood flows to and exits from the heart through large blood vessels called the great vessels.

The heart is divided into a right and left side. Each side contains 2 chambers, called the atrium and the ventricle. They are referred to as the right atrium and right ventricle or the left atrium and left ventricle. The right side receives blood from the body that is depleted of oxygen and full of carbon dioxide. The blood is transported to the heart through the superior and inferior vena cava. The blood is then pumped to the lungs, where the carbon dioxide is removed and oxygen added. This blood is then sent to the left side of the heart, which then pumps it through the aorta to all parts of the body, supplying the oxygen our cells need to function.

The blood is pumped to all organs through vessels called arteries. These arteries branch into smaller vessels, called arterioles, and then capillaries, just like tree limbs divide into smaller and smaller branches that eventually become twigs. The blood returns to the heart through smaller vessels that merge to larger vessels called veins and eventually to the vena cava.

The heart also needs oxygenation, and the arteries that supply it are referred to as the coronary arteries. They too branch into much smaller vessels like the twigs on a tree. The main coronary arteries are the right and left coronary arteries. The right coronary artery (RCA) supplies blood to the right side of the heart. The left coronary artery (LCA) branches into the left anterior descending (LAD) and the circumflex arteries. The LAD supplies blood to the anterior, lateral, and apical portions of the left ventricle while the circumflex sends blood to the left atrium. The LAD is the most commonly occluded artery and the consequences are death or significant impairment.

The heart pumps in a rhythmic fashion. It relaxes to allow blood to enter its chambers and then it squeezes to pump the blood to the lungs and the rest of the body. This must be coordinated, otherwise it won't be able to perform its function. An electrical circuit that is conducted through the heart controls the cadenced heartbeat. The tissue contracts in cycles like the fall of dominoes. If one tissue area beats out of cycle the whole rhythm is thrown off and the heart will malfunction. All of the components must work in synergy to complete the simple task of getting oxygenated blood to all of the tissue and returning de-oxygenated blood to the lungs. If any single constituent part is damaged, then the function of the entire structure will be affected.

Understanding Heart Disease

What is heart disease? How does it occur? What can be done to prevent it? These are the questions that are important to ask and answer to defeat this common killer.

Heart disease encompasses any injury to any structure of the heart. The most common is damage to the coronary arteries from the buildup of plaque in the lining of the vessels. This buildup occurs gradually over time. Eventually the vessels become constricted, limiting blood supply to the heart during times of increased demand. Alternatively, a small clot can cause an acute blockage restricting all blood supply. The result is sudden tissue death, causing acute pain and the potential for death. This is called a myocardial infarction (MI) better known as a heart attack.

The right or left side of the heart can become overworked. This results when a person has untreated high blood pressure or pulmonary hypertension and the heart pumps harder and harder to supply blood to the tissues. The heart muscle initially gets larger over time to accommodate the increased workload. This is called "ventricular hypertrophy." Sometimes the heart muscle is weakened by tissue death that resulted from a MI. Eventually the overworked heart can no longer function as it should. This is known as heart failure. There are many consequences of heart failure; pulmonary edema, liver congestion, low oxygen delivery to the brain and circulatory problems are a few examples.

The conduction system can malfunction, leading to an abnormal rhythm. The rhythm can be too fast or too slow. This is called a "cardiac arrhythmia." Common conduction problems include atrial fibrillation, atrial flutter, supraventricular tachycardia, bradycardia, heart block, ventricular tachycardia, and ventricular fibrillation. Some of these can cause immediate death if the pumping mechanism is affected.

The heart valves can be damaged, resulting in malfunction. They can become too stiff or too floppy. This is called "valvular heart disease," and can result from an acquired congenital defect, damage from an infection, or other causes. The consequence is that too little blood is pumped to the body or lungs or not enough blood is removed from the lungs. This makes the heart work harder to try to meet the body's demands. The damaged valves can also set up blood clot formation, which can lead to sudden death in the form of an embolism or a stroke.

The heart has a clear-cut function, but the processes that require implementation are quite complex. Thus, there are numerous ways in which the heart can malfunction leading to serious problems. The consequences of heart damage are significant and not easily corrected. The key to heart health is prevention or early identification of problems.

The Development of Heart Disease

The term heart disease refers to a whole range of heart problems. This can result from damage to the heart muscles, valves, chambers and blood vessels because of a birth defect or an acquired disorder. Coronary artery disease (CAD), atherosclerotic heart, disease or cardiovascular disease (CVD) refer to damage to the arteries, and it is this arterial damage that causes the bulk of heart disease.

Atherosclerotic heart disease develops over time. Plaque development in the arteries can start as early as adolescence. Factors that contribute to the development of these atherosclerotic plaques and heart disease are many. There are some factors that can't be controlled, such as age and family history. The risk of heart disease increases with age and is greater in those over age 65. Women who have a family history of early onset heart disease and heart attack are at greater risk than those who do not have such a history.

Other risk factors include smoking, obesity, sedentary life style, hypertension, elevated cholesterol, and diabetes. Smoking damages the endothelial cells of the arteries, providing a foundation for the development of plague. Diabetes is also damaging, especially at the level of the microvascular structures making treatment much more difficult. Elevated lipids or cholesterol contribute to the development of the atherosclerotic plaques throughout the arterial system. Uncontrolled hypertension causes the heart to work harder to pump blood through the body, and this overwork leads to failure of the heart muscle over time.

When it comes to heart disease, there are many things that you can do. If you smoke, stop smoking. If you have high cholesterol, hypertension, or diabetes, get the proper medical attention to ensure consistent control of these problems. Regular exercise, proper nutrition, and weight management can help prevent and control these disorders. You have the power to make the difference in your health.

<u>Who develops heart disease?</u>

In 2013, heart disease was responsible for 30 percent of all deaths. Approximately 2,200 people die every day from heart disease and 17 million per year. It is the number one cause of death world-wide.[13]

Even though it is the most common cause of death in men and women, when matched by age, men tend to be at a greater risk. At 40 years of age, the lifetime risk of developing CHD is 49 percent in men and 32 percent in women. The annual incidence is 12 out of 1,000 men and 5 out of 1,000 women. The risk of heart disease increases with age, and for women there is an abrupt increase after menopause. Women lag men by 10- to 20 years when it comes to developing a major consequences of heart disease, such as a heart attack or sudden death.

Even though the mortality rates have decreased by 24 to 50 percent since 1975, in developed countries, some minority groups are still at greater risk of death. The death rates have decreased by 30-60 percent in developed countries but are increasing in developing countries due to the increased life expectancy, adoption of western diets, smoking, and decreased physical activity.

Risk factors for coronary heart disease can be categorized as primary or secondary. Primary factors include a personal history of cardiovascular disease (CVD), elevated lipids, age greater than 55, smoking, diabetes mellitus, hypertension, and a family history of premature CHD. Secondary risk factors include obesity and a sedentary lifestyle.

Anyone with one or more of the above factors should be aware of their increased risk of heart disease and have a low threshold to seek help if they develop any symptoms. Many of the factors can be altered. The damage caused by smoking can be reversed. Controlling blood pressure and diabetes can decrease the chance of unwanted consequences, such as a heart attack. Regular exercise and proper nutrition provide countless benefits in the fight again CHD.

<u>Heart Disease Presentation</u>

The most common symptom of heart disease in both men and women is chest pain. It is typically described as a pressure, heaviness, or tightness, and is sometimes confused with the pain of indigestion. The pain can radiate down the left arm, up the neck, and to the jaw or to the back. It can also be associated with fatigue, shortness of breath, sweating, and nausea. These are the early symptoms of ischemia and if left untreated can lead to a myocardial infarction (MI), also known as a heart attack.

Identifying those suffering from acute coronary syndrome (a term used to describe heart ischemia related to blockage of the coronary arteries) would be easy if the above symptoms were present all the time, but this is not the case. One study showed that of women with a known acute MI, 43 percent did not report chest pain. Of the group, 58 percent reported shortness of breath, 55 percent had weakness, and 43 percent experienced fatigue. In these women, only 30 percent reported early symptoms, indicating ischemia, while the majority had a heart attack on first presentation for care. It is important to note that the early symptoms, which presented more than one month before the heart attack, included unusual fatigue, sleep disturbance, and shortness of breath.

In addition, those presenting with the above symptoms can also be experiencing other problems. The list of other possible diagnoses includes gastroesophageal reflux, stomach ulcer, musculoskeletal pain, and dissection of an aortic aneurysm. Other cardiac-related problems not due to ischemia include: Cardiac Syndrome X, which is a problem with the microvascular of the heart and not the traditional coronary artery obstruction; stress-induced cardiomyopathy, which is caused by intense psychiatric stress; and a spontaneous coronary artery dissection, which is a rare cause of MI not related to coronary artery disease but due to a sudden tear in the artery.

Women tend to have a worse prognosis than men when they develop ischemic heart disease, and in many cases the first presentation may be a heart attack, heart failure, and even sudden death. This is due to a number of reasons. The early symptoms are not necessarily classic for ischemic heart disease and are therefore ignored by the patient and easily misdiagnosed by the healthcare provider. When women seek emergency care for symptoms they are less likely to have an ECG, cardiac monitoring, and cardiac blood tests and are less likely to be seen by a cardiologist for further evaluation. They are most likely to be treated for other non-cardiac related complaints.

Risk factors for heart disease are clear. If you have a personal history of heart disease, a family history of heart disease, smoke, have diabetes, have elevated blood lipids, and are overweight you should be on guard for any of the above symptoms. Even if you don't have any of the above, symptoms of chest pain, shortness of breath, and extreme fatigue should drive you to seek care. If you don't think you are getting an appropriate answer about the cause of your pain, be persistent by either following up with the same doctor or seeking a second opinion. Heart disease is a common killer but early treatment can be lifesaving.

Evaluation of Heart Disease

This is a well-studied problem, and medical science has outlined the pathophysiology, the risk factors, as well as the signs and symptoms. This knowledge has led to the development of effective treatment and preventive strategies. Death from coronary artery disease is preventable in most cases.

The initial evaluation should consist of a complete history and physical examination. This allows the doctor to learn more about your medical history and risk factors. This helps to develop a formal or informal risk assessment. The examination may reveal signs of long-standing problems. Blood tests, chest x-ray (CXR), and electrocardiogram (ECG) are further test that may aide in evaluating your symptoms. The blood test searches for causes of the symptoms and evaluates the health of other organ systems. The CXR can look at the heart size and may show evidence of fluid in the lungs. The ECG shows the electrical activity within the heart and can provide evidence of current or previous heart ischemia or infarction.

Once this initial evaluation is done, further tests may be suggested depending on the results of the above tests and the risk assessment. The exercise stress test is the most common next step. The heart is monitored closely while walking or running on a treadmill. Exercise increases the work of the heart, making the demand for blood supply greater. Partially blocked arteries are unable to deliver on this demand, resulting in ischemia in certain parts of the heart. This ischemia then leads to chest pain, also known as angina.

The exercise stress test has its limitations. Other tests are indicated if a person is unable to exercise or unable to increase the work of the heart. Medications can be given to stress the heart. Radionuclide myocardial imaging, echocardiography, and cardiac computed tomography (CT), either alone or in combination, are alternatives for further evaluating the heart.

Coronary angiography, also called cardiac catheterization, is indicated in the setting of a positive stress test or any other test that is highly suggestive of coronary artery disease. It is the best way to evaluate the coronary arteries. The procedure involves passing a catheter from the femoral artery in the thigh, through the aorta, and into the coronary arteries. A radiolucent dye is injected and video imaging can view the degree of openness of the coronary arteries. This technique also allows for the placement of stents or the injection of thrombolytic medication to break up clots. Ischemic heart disease caused by arterial spasm and micro-vascular disease can't be detected in this manner, which explains why 41 percent of women with signs of ischemic heart disease have a normal cardiac catheterization.

Heart disease is a serious condition and can lead to sudden death and significant morbidity. Tests are available to detect evidence of early disease, providing an opportunity for early treatment, prevention of further damage, and to potentially reverse some damage. Understand your health history so you can know if you are at risk and seek immediate care if you have any symptoms of heart disease. This could be a life-saving step.

Treatment of Heart Disease

A person presenting to the emergency department with symptoms concerning for myocardial infarction (**MI**), also known as a heart attack, are treated in a standard fashion. A history and physical examination are taken quickly while heart monitoring is started and intravenous access is obtained. Blood work and an electrocardiogram (ECG) are done. In most cases, unless there are contraindications, patient is given aspirin immediately. If the blood pressure is high, medications to lower it are prescribed, and this is repeated until a more acceptable range is achieved. Medications to relieve the chest pain are also given. These steps are designed to not only provide comfort but to minimize any further damage to the heart.

The results of the blood test and the ECG will confirm if there is an ongoing acute infarction. The results can even suggest the infarct location within the heart. The next step might include an emergent cardiac catheterization, which would localize the site of the obstructed artery and allow for immediately restoring the flow in the infarcted area by either placing a stent or injecting medication to dissolve the clot. In a small percentage of cases, the angiography might suggest the need for emergency coronary artery bypass surgery.

Once the acute situation has been stabilized, long-term care must be addressed. The goal is to prevent recurrence of the acute ischemia, limit progression of the heart disease, and manage any problems that have developed from the recent event. Common management includes the use of a daily anti-clotting agent, such as aspirin, to decrease the chance of clot development within the atherosclerotic plaques. A beta-blocker is sometimes prescribed to control the heart rate, preventing it from working too hard. Blood pressure control with an angiotensin agent or others is given to also help ease the work of the heart. A statin is given to keep the blood lipid levels within a certain range to prevent further development of atherosclerotic plaques within the arteries. Finally, in those with diabetes, aggressive glucose control is initiated. All of these steps have been proven to decrease the chance of future heart attacks.

A heart attack is a scary event, but also a wake-up call. Treatment is available to manage acute events but it is up to you to be compliant with long-term regimens, otherwise the ischemia will return and eventually cause death. Take advantage of the available medications and listen to the advice of healthcare providers regarding lifestyle changes.

Heart Disease Prevention

Heart disease can present as an acute life-threatening problem or subtly with mild symptoms. Some people are at greater risks than others, but the good news is this: it can be prevented in many cases. Prevention can either be primary, where the causes of heart disease are prevented from occurring, or secondary, where the disease is controlled to prevent the serious consequences of heart disease such as heart attack and sudden death.

Reduction in heart disease prevalence due to risk factor reduction is effective. There was a 31 percent reduction in the incidence of coronary heart disease (CHD) in the period spanning 1992 to 1994 compared to the period of 1980 to 1982. The bulk of the reduction was due to a 41 percent reduction in smoking, and the other due to improved diet. Risk factor reduction is the best way to prevent heart disease. The damage caused by smoking is reversed over time once an individual ceases to smoke. The increased risk caused by smoking is eliminated after 2 to 3 years of cessation. Quitting cigarettes is the most effective step that can be taken to prevent heart disease. Regular exercise, weight control, and proper nutrition are other primary measures that can be taken to prevent the development of CHD.

If you have been diagnosed with hypertension, dyslipidemia, or diabetes, managing your disease is the important first step. Lipid-altering medication has been proven to lead to regression of atherosclerotic changes. Blood pressure control eases the work the heart must do, preventing it from being damaged over time as well as being overworked in an acute crisis. Diabetes control prevents the development of microvascular damage that can lead to premature death from myocardial infarction, stroke, and kidney failure. If these disorders are uncontrolled they can lead to myocardial infarction, sudden death, stroke, and other life-threatening events. There is a wide availability of treatment options to control these common problems.

Heart disease is a prevalent problem but premature death and disability from it can be prevented. The steps outlined above can make the difference between a full healthy life or an early death

Understanding Stroke

Stroke, also known as cerebrovascular accident (CVA), is the second most common cause of death worldwide and the third to cancer at 22.8 percent and heart disease contributing to 28.5 percent. This is a common problem, which can affect anyone but becomes more prevalent with age.[13]

Stroke is an acute neurologic injury that occurs because of diminished oxygen supply to areas of the brain. Usually it is to one specific area but the entire brain can be affected. The most common type of stroke is the ischemic type, representing 80 percent of all strokes while hemorrhagic strokes occur 20 percent of the time. An ischemic stroke results when there is a sudden obstruction of blood supply, usually due to a thrombus or embolism lodged in a blood vessel. A hemorrhagic stroke occurs when there is a sudden bleed, either in the brain or in the subarachnoid space, into the cerebrovascular fluid (CSF) surrounding the brain.

The symptoms of a stroke may vary depending on the location within the brain, severity of the stroke and type of stroke. In general, symptoms of sudden asymmetrical weakness, difficulty speaking, facial drooping, or blindness are highly concerning for an acute stroke. Other symptoms can include memory loss, headache, nausea, vomiting, and fainting. There is a special case of stroke in which the neurologic deficits are reversible. This is called a TIA (Transient Ischemic Attack). The symptoms usually resolve in less than 24 hours.

The prognosis of stroke is dependent upon many factors, but age is the primary predictor of outcome. Those greater than age 65 have a much higher risk of dying within 2 months of the event. The other factor is the type of stroke. The 30-day fatality rate for an ischemic stroke is 16 to 23 percent while the rate is much higher in those who experience a hemorrhagic stroke. Other predictors include severity of neurologic deficit, volume of brain involvement as determined by imaging studies, acute interventions, and post-stroke rehabilitation care.

One large study examined the residual neurologic deficits still present after 6 months in those over 65 years of age. Fifty percent had weakness on one side of the body, 46 percent had cognitive deficits, 20 percent experienced visual field deficits, 19 percent had aphasia (disturbance in comprehension and formulation of language) and 15 percent had sensory deficits. Approximately more than 30 percent experienced depression and were unable to have social independence, while more than 25 percent were institutionalized. In addition to the above, stroke victims are at risk of other medical complications and interventions. They may require intubation and mechanical ventilation if the stroke involves the area of the brain that controls respiration. They are at higher risk of acquiring pneumonia, experiencing falls, having cardiac arrest, and developing thromboembolic events such as pulmonary emboli or deep venous thrombosis. Even the treatment of stroke can lead to medical complications, such as a gastrointestinal bleeding from thrombolytic agents used to treat ischemic strokes.

Stroke or CVA is a common event with a high mortality rate and can lead to significant morbidity. The signs and symptoms are well defined and the key to complete recuperation and survival is early recognition and timely intervention. You should seek immediate care if you or someone you know experiences symptoms of a stroke.

Ischemic Stroke

An ischemic stroke occurs when the blood supply to a region of the brain is blocked resulting in tissue death. It is the cause of 80 percent of all strokes. The causes of the ischemia are variable but atherosclerosis (plaque build-up in the arteries) is a major contributor. It is important to identify the causes of a stroke to appropriately manage the current incident and to prevent recurrence.

In an ischemic stroke blood flow to the brain is compromised. There are many potential causes, but the most common subtypes include thrombotic, embolic, and hypoperfusion. Thrombotic strokes can result when a thrombus or clot forms within an artery, blocking blood flow. An embolic stroke can occur when a small clot travels from a distant location and finally lodges in a small artery blocking blood flow. Finally, hypoperfusion occurs when there is a traumatic event to the body that prevents blood from being pumped to the brain. If blood flow is not restored within minutes, neurologic injury will occur. Examples of hypoperfusion events include cardiac arrest, hypovolemic shock from large blood loss, cardiac arrhythmia, and a large pulmonary embolus.

In a thrombotic or embolic stroke, a blocked artery diminishes or completely obstructs blood supply to a region of the brain. The tissue becomes pale and, after several hours to days, the tissue becomes congested with dilated blood vessels and small areas of minute bleeding. If the blood flow is restored, either because of the clot migrating or dissolving, then the returned blood flow can leak into the brain tissue, causing a larger hemorrhage and greater problems.

Thrombotic strokes can occur in large or small vessels. Arteriosclerosis, arterial dissection, arteritis, and fibromuscular dysplasia are conditions that increase the likelihood of this occurring. Small vessels can also undergo vasoconstriction, producing diminished blood supply. Individuals with conditions that make them more likely to clot are also at greater risk. Conditions such as Factor V Leiden, Protein S, and Protein C deficiencies are examples. Other conditions, such as Sickle Cell Anemia and Polycythemia Vera also predispose a sufferer to clotting. Small vessel strokes can also occur in the setting of hypertension or with age. The tissue affected is in small areas of the brain, and the symptoms can go unnoticed until there is an accumulation of damage. These are called lacunar infarcts.

Embolic stroke occurs because of a problem in another part of the body. A small clot peels away from its source, traveling to the brain to obstruct an artery there. The embolism can come from plaque formation in the aorta or carotid artery or they can come from embolism forming on the heart valves. In some cases, the source is never found. Common conditions that can form emboli include myocardial infarction, a defect heart valve, a mechanical heart valve, an infected heart valve, atrial fibrillation, cardiomyopathy, and a carotid artery or aortic plaque.

Ischemic strokes are a major cause of death and disability, especially in the elderly. Early intervention is the key to survival and understanding the risk factors can aide in prevention. Seek care immediately if you or someone you know experiences the symptoms of a stroke.

<u>Hemorrhagic Stroke</u>

Hemorrhagic strokes represent 20 percent of all cerebrovascular accidents (CVA). The presentation and management are different than an ischemic stroke and the prognosis is much worse. There are 2 types of hemorrhagic stroke: intracerebral and subarachnoid.

Intracerebral hemorrhage results from bleeding within the brain tissue, which usually starts in the small arteries. As the bleeding grows it spreads around the brain and causes a hematoma. The hematoma may stabilize and eventually resolve on its own. The greatest concern occurs when the bleeding continues, causing a larger hematoma. As the hematoma grows it damages the brain by compressing the surrounding tissue causing swelling.

The presenting symptoms are based on the region of the brain affected, but they can go undetected for some time. The symptoms may include weakness, problems walking, and difficulty speaking. As the hematoma grows it can cause headaches, nausea, vomiting, and loss of consciousness. The most common cause of this type of stroke includes hypertension, trauma, and rupture of a vascular malformation. This is also more likely to occur in illicit drug users and those with a bleeding tendency. Other less common causes include bleeding from a tumor, a ruptured aneurysm, and vasculitis (an inflammatory condition of the blood vessels).

A subarachnoid hemorrhage occurs with sudden acute bleeding into the fluid surrounding the brain and spinal cord within the subarachnoid space that surrounds the brain. A large amount of blood in the cerebrospinal fluid increases the pressure within this delicately balanced area. This increased pressure can cause a shift in the brain structures. Edema usually develops. This shift in the structures and associated edema will compromise neurologic function if prompt treatment is not given.

The amount of blood loss is usually large, contributing to a sudden onset of symptoms such as headache, fainting, memory loss, and vomiting. The phrase "worse headache of my life" is commonly used to describe the severity of the pain. This type of bleeding usually results from a ruptured aneurysm or some other type of vascular malformation and represents a life-threatening emergency. If left untreated, death or coma can occur rapidly.

Symptoms of sudden severe headache, especially associated with vomiting and loss of consciousness require prompt medical care. Even though there are many other potential causes, a hemorrhagic stroke is the one that needs to be considered first. Health care providers only have a short period of time to intervene to save the affected person. If you or someone you know, experiences these symptoms, seek care immediately.

THE BOTTOM LINE

- After a certain age women are at risk for medical problems such as hypertension, diabetes, heart disease and stroke.
- A heart attack or a stroke is a major-medical emergency and time is of essence in getting treated.
- Getting appropriate emergency care as quickly as possible can be life-saving.

Conclusion

This book has been more than ten years in the making. My reasons for writing this guide have remained the same since I began the first chapter. There is so much a woman needs to know about her body in order to prevent problems and manage common health conditions. Over the years, I have tried to educate my patients, but of course this is impossible to do in a comprehensive manner during a short office visit. *The Essence of You* is my attempt to put all this information in one place. This book is a resource that can be referred to repeatedly over the years and even shared with friends and family. Please remember this is a guide designed to give you knowledge so that you can work more productively with your healthcare provider to maintain good health.

References

[1] Understanding the Health Literacy of America Results of the National Assessment of Adult Literacy. Carolyn Crane Cutilli, MSN, RN, ONC, CRRN and Ian M. Bennett, MD, PhD Orthop Nurs. 2009; 28(1): 27–34.

[2] Women as health care decision-makers: implications for health care coverage in the United States. Matoff-Stepp S, Applebaum B, Pooler J, Kavanagh E. J Health Care Poor Underserved. 2014 Nov;25(4):1507-13.

Chapter 1

[1] Novak's Gynecology. 13th edition. Jonathan S. Berek, editor. Lippincott Williams & Wilkins 2002. Chapter 5 Anatomy and Embryology and Chapter 7 Reproductive Physiology.

[2] Gray's Anatomy. 30th edition. Carmine D. Clemente, editor. Lea&Febiger. 1985.

[3] Clinical Gynecologic Endocrinology and Infertility. 5th Edition. Leon Speroff, Robert H. Glass and Nathan G. Kase. Williams & Wilkins 1994. Part I: Reproductive Physiology.

Chapter 2

[1] Novak's Gynecology. 13th edition. Jonathan S. Berek, editor. Lippincott Williams & Wilkins 2002. Chapter 23 Puberty.

2   Clinical Gynecologic Endocrinology and Infertility. 5th Edition. Leon Speroff, Robert H. Glass and Nathan G. Kase. Williams & Wilkins 1994. Part II: Clinical Endocrinology.

3   Prevalence and Characteristics of Sexual Violence, Stalking, and Intimate Partner Violence Victimization — National Intimate Partner and Sexual Violence Survey, United States, 2011 Surveillance Summaries September 5, 2014 / 63(SS08);1-18. CDC Morbidity and Mortality Weekly Report.

4   Sexual Violence in Youth. Findings from the 2012 National Intimate Partner and Sexual Violence Survey. National Center for Injury Prevention and Control. CDC.gov.

Chapter 3

1   Lowy, DR. and Schiller JT. Prophylactic human papillomavirus vaccines. The Journal of Clinical Investigation. Volume 116, May 2006, 1167-1173.

2   Spitzer, Mark, Gold, Michael and Cox, J. Thomas. New Options in HPV Prevention. Supplement to OBG Management. July 2006, S2-22.

3   Vaccinate Women. A periodical for obstetrician/gynecologists from the immunization action coalition. Volume 5-Number1. August 2006

4   Sulak PJ, Scow RD, Preece C, Riggs MW, and Kuehl TJ. Hormone Withdrawal Symptoms in Oral Contraceptive Users. Obstetrics & Gynecology Vol 95, No. 2, February 2000.

5   Contraceptive Technology, 18th Edition. Hatcher, RA, Trussell, J, Stewart F, Nelson AL, Gates W, Guest F, and Kowal D. Ardent Media, Inc. New York 2004.

6   Premenstrual Syndrome. ACOG Practice Bulletin. Number 15, April 2000. 917-24.

7   Yonkers, Kimberly A. Management Strategies for PMS/PMDD. The Journal of Family Practice. Supplement. September 2004. S15-20.

8   Girman, A., Lee, R., and Kligler, B. An Integrative Medicine Approach to Premenstrual Syndrome. Am J Obstet Gynecol. Volume 188, Number 5. S56-65.

9   Management of Anovulatory Bleeding. ACOG Practice Bulletin. Number 14, March 2000. 434-441.

10 Richard L. Sweet and Ronald S. Gibbs. Infectious Diseases of the Female Genital Tract. 3rd edition 1995 Williams & Wilkins

11 Recurrent Urinary Tract Infection in Women: Emerging Concepts Regarding Etiology and Treatment Considerations. E. Ann Gormley. Current Urology Reports 2003, 4:399-403

Chapter 4 and 5

1   Giraldo P, von Nowaskonski A, Gomes FA, Linhares I, Neves NA, Witkin SS. Vaginal colonization by Candida in asymptomatic women with and without a history of recurrent vulvovaginal candidiasis. Obstet Gynecol. 2000 Mar;95(3):413-6.

2   Horowitz BJ, Edelstein SW, Lippman L. tropicalis vulvovaginitis. Obstet Gynecol. 1985 Aug;66(2):229-32

3   Thomason JL, Gelbart SM. Trichomonas vaginalis. Obstet Gynecol. 1989 Sep;74(3 Pt 2):536-41.

4   Vaginitis. ACOG Practice Bulletin. Clinical Management Guideline. #72. 2006. Reaffirmed 2011.

5   DeWaay DJ, Syrop CH, Nygaard IE, Davis WA, and Van Voorhis BJ. Natural History of Uterine Polyps and Leiomyomata. Obstet Gynecol 2002;100:3-7.

6   Stewart EA and Morton CC. The Genetics of Uterine Leiomyomata. Obstet Gynecol 2006;107:917-921.

7   Steinauer J, Pritts EA, Jackson R, and Jacoby AF. Systematic Review of Mifepristone for the Treatment of Uterine Leiomyomata Obstet Gynecol 2004;103:1331-36.

8   Surgical Alternatives to Hysterectomy in the Management of Leiomyomas. ACOG Practice Bulletin. May 2000; 16:665-687.

9   Raja A. Sayegh. Uterine Fibroids: The Most Common Benign Tumors of the Female Reproductive Tract. AstraZeneca Gynecology Diploma Program. December 2013.

[10] Marsh EE, Ekpo GE, Cardozo ER, Brocks M, Dune T, Cohen LS. Racial differences in fibroid prevalence and ultrasound findings in asymptomatic young women (18-30 years old): a pilot study. Fertil Steril. 2013 Jun;99(7):1951-7.

[11] Baird DD, Dunson DB, Hill MC, Cousins D, Schectman JM. High cumulative incidence of uterine leiomyoma in black and white women: ultrasound evidence. Am J Obstet Gynecol. 2003 Jan;188(1):100-7.

[12] Spies JB[1], Myers ER, Worthington-Kirsch R, Mulgund J, Goodwin S, Mauro M; FIBROID Registry Investigators.The FIBROID Registry: symptom and quality-of-life status 1 year after therapy. Obstet Gynecol. 2005 Dec;106(6):1309-18

[13] ACOG Committee on Practice Bulletins. ACOG practice bulletin. Medical management of endometriosis. Number 11, December 1999. Int J Gynaecol Obstet. 2000 Nov;71(2):183-96

[14] Sutton CJ[1], Pooley AS, Ewen SP, Haines P. Follow-up report on a randomized controlled trial of laser laparoscopy in the treatment of pelvic pain associated with minimal to moderate endometriosis. Fertil Steril. 1997 Dec;68(6):1070-4

[15] http://www.4women.gov/faq/ovarian_cysts.htm Ovarian cyst

[16] Management of Adnexal Masses. ACOG Practice Bulletin. Number 83, July 2007, reaffirmed 2013.

[17] Is Prior Uterine Surgery a Risk Factor for Adenomyosis? Panganamamula U, et al. Obstetrics & Gynecology. 2004; 104:1034-8.

[18] Adenomyosis and subfertility: a systematic review of prevalence, diagnosis, treatment and fertility outcomes. Maheshwari A., et al. Human Reproduction Update, Vol 18, No. 4, 2012; 374-392.

[19] James Trussell, PhD. Contraceptive failure in the United States. Contraception. 2011 May; 83(5): 397–404.

[20] Long-Active Reversible Contraception: Implants and Intrauterine Devices. The American College of Obstetricians and Gynecologists, Practice Bulletin, Number 121. July 2011. Reaffirmed 2013.

[21] Cooper JM[1], Carignan CS, Cher D, Kerin JF; Selective Tubal Occlusion Procedure 2000 Investigators Group. Microinsert nonincisional hysteroscopic sterilization. Obstet Gynecol. 2003 Jul;102(1):59-67.

22   Peterson HB. Sterilization. Obstet Gynecol. 2008 Jan;111(1):189-203

23   Guttmacher AF. Factors affecting normal expectancy of conception. J Am Med Assoc 1956;161:885.

24   Anjani Chandra, Ph.D., and Casey E. Copen, Ph.D., National Center for Health Statistics; and Elizabeth Hervey Stephen, Ph.D., Georgetown University. Infertility and impaired fecundity in the United States, 1982-2010; Data from the National Survey of Family Growth. National Health Statistics Reports. Number 67 August 14, 2013.

Chapter 6

1   Premenstrual Syndrome. ACOG Practice Bulletin. Number 15, April 2000. 917-24.

2   Yonkers, Kimberly A. Management Strategies for PMS/PMDD. The Journal of Family Practice. Supplement. September 2004. S15-20.

3   Girman, A., Lee, R., and Kligler, B. An Integrative Medicine Approach to Premenstrual Syndrome. Am J Obstet Gynecol. Volume 188, Number 5. S56-65.

4   American College of Obstetricians and Gynecologists Practice Bulletin. Diagnosis of Abnormal Uterine Bleeding in Reproductive-Aged Women. Clinical Management Guidelines. Number 128, July 2012.

5   Transobturator Tape Compared with Tension-Free Vaginal Tape for the Treatment of Stress Urinary Incontinence *A Randomized Controlled Trial.* Obstetrics & Gynecology. Vol. 111, No. 3, March 2008

6   Retropubic versus Transobturator Midurethral Slings for Stress Incontinence. Urinary Continence Treatment Network. N Engl J Med 362;22 June 3, 2010

7   Stress urinary incontinence in women: Choosing a primary surgical procedure. UpToDate Jan 2014

8   Stress urinary incontinence in women: Persistent/recurrent symptoms after surgical treatment. UpToDate Jan 2014

9   Stress urinary incontinence in women: Transobturator midurethral slings. UpToDate Jan 2014

[10] Stress urinary incontinence in women: Retropubic midurethral slings. UpToDate Feb 2013.

[11] CDC.gov. Overweight and Obesity Facts http://www.cdc.gov/obesity/data/adult.html

[12] Cynthia L. Ogden, PhD; Margaret D. Carroll, MSPH; Brian K. Kit, MD, MPH; Katherine M. Flegal, PhD. Prevalence of Childhood and Adult Obesity in the United States, 2011-2012 *JAMA*. 2014;311(8):806-814. doi:10.1001/jama.2014.732.

[13] UpToDate: Etiology and natural history of obesity. October 26, 2012.

[14] UpToDate: Obesity in Adults: Drug Therapy. Oct 16, 2014.

[15] Surgery for Obesity. Colquitt JL, Picot J, Loveman E, Clegg AJ. The Cochrane Collaboration. The Cochrane Library. 2009 Issue2.

Chapter 7

[1] Shanafelt TD, Barton DL, Adjei AA, Loprinzi CL. Pathophysiology and Treatment of Hot Flashes. Mayo Clin Proc. 2002; 77:1207-1218.

[2] Freedman RR. Current Best Treatments for Hot Flashes. Menopause Management. Nov/Dec 2006 20-25.

[3] Gordon PR, Kerwin JP, Boesen KG, Senf J. Sertraline to treat hot flashes: a randomized controlled, double-blind, crossover trial in a general population. Menopause 2006; 13:568-575.

[4] Pandya KJ, Morrow GR, Roscoe JA, Zhao K, Hickok JT, Pajan E, Sweeney TJ, Banaerjee TK, Flynn PJ. Gabapentin for hot flashes in 420 women with breast cancer: a randomized double-blind placebo-controlled study. Lancet 2005;366:818.

[5] Swanson SG, Drosman S, Helmond FA, Stathopoulos VM. Tibolone for the treatment of moderate to severe vasomotor symptoms and genital atrophy in postmenopausal women: a multicenter, randomized, double-blind, placebo-controlled study. Menopause 2006; 13:917-925

[6] Christopher I. Li, MD, PhD; Kathleen E. Malone, PhD; Peggy L. Porter, MD; et al. Relationship Between Long Durations and Different Regimens of Hormone Therapy and Risk of Breast Cancer. JAMA. 2003;289(24):3254-3263.

[7] <u>Writing Group for the Women's Health Initiative Investigators</u>. Risks and Benefits of Estrogen Plus Progestin in Healthy Postmenopausal Women: Principal Results From the Women's Health Initiative Randomized Controlled Trial. JAMA. 2002;288(3):321-333

[8] Delaney MF. Strategies for the prevention and treatment of osteoporosis during early postmenopause. American Journal of Obstetrics and Gynecology (2006) 194, S12-23.

[9] Sambrook P. and Cooper C. Osteoporosis. The Lancet. June 2006. Vol 367 2010-2018.

[10] Miller RG. Osteoporosis in postmenopausal women: Therapy options across a wide range of risk for fracture. Geriatrics. January 2006 Volume 61, Number 1. 24-30.

[11] Lane NE. Epidemiology, etiology, and diagnosis of osteoporosis. American Journal of Obstetrics & Gynecology. (2006) 194, S3-11.

[12] Rosen CJ and Brown SA. A rational approach to evidence gaps in the management of osteoporosis. The American Journal of Medicine. (2005) 118, 1183-1189.

[13] Bonnick SL and Shulman L. Monitoring Osteoporosis Therapy: Bone Mineral Density, Bone Turnover Markers, or Both? The American Journal of Medicine (2006) Vol 119 (4A), 25S-31S.

Chapter 8

[1] National Highway Traffic Safety Administration. Final regulatory impact analysis amendment to Federal Motor Vehicle Safety Standard 208. Passenger car front seat occupant protection. Washington, DC: US Department of Transportation, National Highway Traffic Safety Administration; 1984. Publication no. DOT-HS-806-572. Available at http://www-nrd.nhtsa.dot.gov/pubs/806572.pdf. Accessed September 8, 2014.1

[2] Ladau, Kristina. "What is Nutrition?" *www.whatisnutritiontips.com*. Ed. Kristina Ladau. What is nutrition? Tips for Living Well, n.d. Web. 11 Nov. 2014.

3   Nordqvist, Christian. "What is healthy eating? What is a good diet?" *MNT Knowledge Center.* MediLexicon International, 9 Sept. 2014. Web. 11 Nov. 2014. <http://www.medicalnewstoday.com/articles/153998.php>.

4   Preventable Deaths: CDC.gov/media/releases/2014/p0501 Press Release: Up to 40 percent of annual deaths from each of five leading US causes are preventable.

5   Staff, Mayo Clinic. "Healthy Lifestyle Nutrition and healthy eating." *Mayo Clinic.* N.p., n.d. Web. 11 Nov. 2014

6   Thomson, Janet. *28 Days To A Better Body.* Allentown: People's Medical Society, 1996. 5. Print.

7   Importance of Water in the Diet. *CRUISING CHEMISTRY An introduction to the World Around You.* Ed. Dr. Diane Szaflarski, Dr. Robert Dean, and Dr. Melanie Dean. N.p., n.d. Web. 16 Nov. 2014. <http://people.chem.duke.edu/~jds/cruise_chem/water/watdiet.html>.

8   "Best Overall Diets." *U.S. News & World Report HEALTH.* U.S.News & World Report, n.d. Web. 16 Nov. 2014. <http://health.usnews.com/best-diet/best-overall-diets?page=4>.

9   Mechanism of nutrient absorption and malabsorption. UpToDate March 21, 2013.

10 Healthy diet in Adults. UpToDate. Jan 08, 2015

11 Dietary Carbohydrates. UpToDate. Nov 19, 2014.

12 12. Nutrition for Everyone: Protein. www.cdc.gov.

13 The Nutrition Source. Fiber. Harvard T.H.Chan School of Public Health.

14 http://www.healthline.com/health-slideshow/understanding-glycemic-index#1

15 http://www.calorieking.com/

16 http://www.msn.com/en-us/health/fitness

17 http://www.womenshealthmag.com/

18 http://www.mendosa.com/gi.htm

19 http://www.nhs.uk/Livewell/fitness/Pages/Whybeactive.aspx. accessed July 6, 2016

20 http://www.hopkinsmedicine.org/health/healthy_heart/move_more/ three-kinds-of-exercise-that-boost-heart-health. accessed July 6, 2016

21 http://www.heart.org/HEARTORG/HealthyLiving/Physical Activity/FitnessBasics/Types-of-Fitness_UCM_462352_Article.jsp#. V2j5nE1f2po. accessed July 6, 2016

22 https://www.cdc.gov/physicalactivity/. accessed July 6, 2016

23 http://smokefree.gov/health-effects

24 Benefits and Risks of Smoking Cessation. UpToDate. Feb 2015

25 American Lung Association: What's in a Cigarette. http://www.lung. org/stop-smoking/smoking-facts/whats-in-a-cigarette

26 American Cancer Society: How many people use tobacco? http:// www.cancer.org/cancer/cancercauses/tobaccocancer/questionsabout smokingtobaccoandhealth/questions-about-smoking-tobacco-and- health-how-many-use

27 Alcohol Effects on the Body. https://www.niaaa.nih.gov/alcohol- health/alcohols-effects-body. July 9, 2016.

28 Alcohol Use Disorder. http://bestpractice.bmj.com/best-practice/ monograph/198.html. July 9, 2016.

29 https://www.niaaa.nih.gov/alcohol-health/overview-alcohol- consumption/alcohol-use-disorders. July 11, 2016.

30 http://www.cdc.gov/alcohol/index.htm July 15, 2016.

Chapter 9

1 Siegel RL, Miller KD, Jemal A. Cancer Statistics, 2016. CA Cancer J Clin. 2016 Jan-Feb;66(1):7-30.

2 Howlader N, Noone AM, Krapcho M, Miller D, Bishop K, Altekruse SF, Kosary CL, Yu M, Ruhl J, Tatalovich Z, Mariotto A, Lewis DR, Chen HS, Feuer EJ, Cronin KA (eds). SEER Cancer Statistics Review, 1975-2013, National Cancer Institute. Bethesda, MD, http:// seer.cancer.gov/csr/1975_2013/, based on November 2015 SEER data submission, posted to the SEER web site, April 2016.

3 Gail MH, Brinton LA, Byar DP, Corle DK, Green SB, Shairer C, Mulvihill JJ: Projecting individualized probabilities of developing

breast cancer for white females who are being examined annually. J Natl Cancer Inst 81(24):1879-86, 1989.

[4] Hendrick RE, Helvie MA. Mammography screening: a new estimate of number needed to screen to prevent one breast cancer death. AJR Am J Roentgenol. 2012 Mar;198(3):723-8.

[5] http://www.cancer.org/cancer/breastcancer/moreinformation/breast cancerearlydetection/index. Accessed December 27, 2016.

[6] Cuzick J et al. Tamoxifen for prevention of breast cancer: extended long-term follow-up of the IBIS-I breast cancer prevention trial. Lancet Oncol. 2015 Jan;16(1):67-75.

[7] Nelson HD, Smith ME, Griffin JC, Fu R. Use of medications to reduce risk for primary breast cancer: a systematic review for the U.S. Preventive Services Task Force. Ann Intern Med. 2013 Apr 16;158(8):604-14.

[8] Antoniou A, et al. Average risks of breast and ovarian cancer associated with BRCA1 or BRCA2mutations detected in case Series unselected for family history: a combined analysis of 22 studies. Am J Hum Genet. 2003 May;72(5):1117-30.

[9] Domchek SM et al. Association of risk-reducing surgery in BRCA1 or BRCA2 mutation carriers with cancer risk and mortality. JAMA. 2010 Sep 1;304(9):967-75.

[10] Iodice S, Barile M, Rotmensz N, Feroce I, Bonanni B, Radice P, Bernard L, Maisonneuve P, Gandini S. Oral contraceptive use and breast or ovarian cancer risk in BRCA1/2 carriers: a meta-analysis. Eur J Cancer. 2010 Aug;46(12):2275-84.

[11] Torre LA, Bray F, Siegel RL, Ferlay J, Lortet-Tieulent J, Jemal A. Global cancer statistics, 2012. CA Cancer J Clin. 2015 Mar;65(2):87-10

[12] https://www.cancer.gov/about-cancer/causes-prevention/risk/ infectious-agents/hpv-fact-sheet.

[13] Muñoz N, Bosch FX, de Sanjosé S, Herrero R, Castellsagué X, Shah KV, Snijders PJ, Meijer CJ; International Agency for Research on Cancer Multicenter Cervical Cancer Study Group. Epidemiologic classification of human papillomavirus types associated with cervical cancer. N Engl J Med. 2003 Feb 6;348(6):518-27.

[14] https://www.cancer.gov/about-cancer/causes-prevention/risk/infectious-agents/hpv-vaccine-fact-sheet

[15] J Thomas Cox, Joel M Palefsky. Recommendations for the use of human papillomavirus vaccines. UpToDate. Updated Nov 29, 2016.

[16] Bokhman JV. Two pathogenetic types of endometrial carcinoma. Gynecol Oncol. 1983 Feb;15(1):10-7.

[17] Chen LM and Berek JS. Endometrial carcinoma: Clinical features and diagnosis. UpToDate. June 6, 2016.

[18] Judson PL, Habermann EB, Baxter NN, Durham SB, Virnig BA. Trends in the incidence of invasive and in situ vulvar carcinoma. Obstet Gynecol. 2006 May;107(5):1018-22.

[19] ACOG Committee Opinion No. 675: Management of vulvar intraepithelial neoplasia. Committee on Gynecologic Practice of American College Obstetricians and Gynecologists. Obstet Gynecol. 2016 Oct;128(4).

[20] van Seters M, van Beurden M, de Craen AJ. Is the assumed natural history of vulvar intraepithelial neoplasia III based on enough evidence? A systematic review of 3322 published patients. Gynecol Oncol. 2005 May;97(2):645-51.

[21] Campion MJ, Greenberg MD, Kazamel TI. Clinical manifestations and natural history of genital human papillomavirus infections. Obstet Gynecol Clin North Am. 1996 Dec;23(4):783-809.

[22] Shah CA, Goff BA, Lowe K, Peters WA 3rd, Li CI. Factors affecting risk of mortality in women with vaginal cancer. Obstet Gynecol. 2009 May;113(5):1038-45.

[23] Novak's Gynecology. 13th edition. Jonathan S. Berek, editor. Lippincott Williams & Wilkins 2002. Section VI- Gynecologic Oncology.

[24] https://www.cdc.gov/cancer/ovarian/statistics/. Accessed Dec 29, 2016.

[25] Collaborative Group on Epidemiological Studies of Ovarian Cancer. Ovarian cancer and oral contraceptives: collaborative reanalysis of data from 45 epidemiological studies including 23,257 women with ovarian cancer and 87,303 controls. Lancet. 2008 Jan 26;371(9609):303-14.

Chapter 10

[1] Kepenekci I et al. Prevalence of Pelvic Floor Disorders in the Female Population and the Impact of Age, Mode of Delivery, and Parity. Dis Colon Rectum 2011;54:85-94.

[2] Wu JM et al. Prevalence and Trends of Symptomatic Pelvic Floor Disorders in U.S. Women. Obstet Gynecol. 2014 January; 123(1) 141-148.

[3] Nygaard I, Barber MD, Burgio KL, Kenton K, Meikle S, Schaffer J, et al. Prevalence of symptomatic pelvic floor disorders in US women. Jama. 2008;300(11):1311-6.

[4] Handa VL, Blomquist JL, Knoepp LR, Hoskey KA, McDermott KC, Muñoz A. Pelvic Floor Disorders 5–10 Years After Vaginal or Cesarean Childbirth. Obstetrics & Gynecology. 2011;118(4):777-84.

[5] Chantale Dumoulin, E. Jean C Hay-Smith and Gabrielle Mac Habée-Séguin. Pelvic floor muscle training versus no treatment, or inactive control treatments, for urinary incontinence in women. Cochrane Database Syst Rev. 2014 May 14;(5):CD005654.

[6] Jonsson Funk M, Siddiqui NY, Kawasaki A, Wu JM. Long-term outcomes after stress urinary incontinence surgery. Obstet Gynecol 2012 Jul;120(1):83-90.

[7] Jennifer M. Wu, Catherine A. Matthews, Mitchell M. Conover, Virginia Pate, Michele Jonsson Funk. Lifetime Risk of Stress Incontinence or Pelvic Organ Prolapse Surgery. Obstet Gynecol. 2014 Jun; 123(6): 1201–1206.

[8] Victor W. Nitti, MD. Complications of midurethral slings and their management. Can Urol Assoc J. 2012 Oct; 6(5 Suppl 2): S120–S122.

[9] Ulmsten U. An introduction to tension-free vaginal tape (TVT)--a new surgical procedure for treatment of female urinary incontinence. Int Urogynecol J Pelvic Floor Dysfunct. 2001;12 Suppl 2: S3-4.

[10] Renu S Eapen and Sidney B Radomski. Review of the epidemiology of overactive bladder. Res Rep Urol. 2016; 8: 71–76.

Chapter 11

1   Egan BM, Zhao Y, Axon RN. US trends in prevalence, awareness, treatment, and control of hypertension, 1988-2008. JAMA. 2010 May 26;303(20):2043-50.

2   Mark A. Garber and Matthew L. Lanternier. The Family Practice Handbook. University of Iowa. 4th edition Mosby 2001. pg 100-102.

3   Wang TJ, Vasan RS. Epidemiology of uncontrolled hypertension in the United States. Circulation. 2005 Sep 13;112(11):1651-62.

4   Isselbacher, Braunwald, Wilson, Martin, Fauci, and Kasper, editors. Harrison's Principles of Internal Medicine. Companion Handbook. 13th Edition McGraw-Hill Inc. 1995. Pg 340-46.

5   http://www.heart.org/HEARTORG/Conditions/HighBlood Pressure/PreventionTreatmentofHighBloodPressure/Types-of-Blood-Pressure-Medications. Accessed January 2017.

6   Menke A, Casagrande S, Geiss L, Cowie CC. Prevalence of and Trends in Diabetes Among Adults in the United States, 1988-2012. JAMA. 2015 Sep 8;314(10):1021-9.

7   http://www.diabetes.org/diabetes-basics/statistics/ Accessed January 2017.

8   Dabelea D et al. Prevalence of type 1 and type 2 diabetes among children and adolescents from 2001 to 2009. JAMA. 2014 May 7;311(17):1778-86.

9   McCulloch DK, Robertson RP. Risk factors for type 2 diabetes mellitus. UpToDate. May 09, 2016.

10 McCulloch DK, Robertson RP. Pathogenesis of type 2 diabetes mellitus. UpToDate. Nov 17, 2016.

11 Diabetes Prevention Program. National Diabetes Information Clearinghouse. NIDDK. NIH.

12 Clemente, Carmine D. Gray's Anatomy 30th American Edition 621-645. Lea&Febiger Philadelphia.

13 AHA Statistical Update. Heart Disease and Stroke Statistics-2016 Update. Circulation. 2016;133:e38-e360. Originally published December 16, 2015.

[14] The American Heart Association. Heart Disease, Stroke and Research Statistics 2016. http://www.americanheart.org/.

[15] American College of Cardiology http://www.acc.org/

[16] Etiology and classification of stroke. UpToDate May 2013

Acknowledgments

Producing a book of this nature comes with some sacrifices and this is usually shared by family. I owe a debt of gratitude to my husband and children for their undying support. My husband's endless encouragement and eternal confidence in my abilities has kept me going. My amazing children are a constant source of inspiration and I live to make them proud. I would like to thank my editor, Charlene Giannetti, for her patience and attention to detail as we worked to make this book ready for publication. I would also like to thank Marti Sichel, my copy editor, for her meticulous review and sincere suggestions aimed at making this book inclusive.

About the Author

Denise Howard attended the University of Mississippi and received her Medical Degree and Masters in Public Health from the Johns Hopkins University in Baltimore, Maryland. She completed her residency at Magee-Womens Hospital, University of Pittsburgh Medical Center, and a fellowship in Urogynecology and Reconstructive Pelvic Surgery at the University of Michigan Health System where she also served on the faculty. Her practice, first in Georgia and then in Abu Dhabi and Doha in the Middle East, has focused on Obstetrics, Gynecology, and Gynecologic surgery. Currently, she is a Senior Attending Physician at Sidra Medical and Research Center and an Assistant Professor of Clinical Obstetrics and Gynecology, Weill Cornell Medicine-Qatar, where she teaches and mentors medical students.

Index

---

www.ingramcontent.com/pod-product-compliance
Lightning Source LLC
Chambersburg PA
CBHW022053210326
41519CB00054B/334